The Normalization of the HIV and AIDS Epidemic in South Africa

This book explores the normalization of HIV and AIDS, reflecting upon the intended and unintended consequences of the multifarious "AIDS industry."

The Normalization of the HIV and AIDS Epidemic in South Africa deals with the manner in which the HIV and AIDS epidemic has become such a well-known disease with such wide-ranging ramifications. With its focus on the "AIDS industry," this book examines issues such as the framing of the HIV and AIDS epidemic in a manner that greatly fostered notions of stigmatization and moralization. This book looks at the complexities of dealing with the epidemic in contemporary South Africa, examining the difficulties of addressing the social aspects of a disease in the context of increased focus on technological quick-fix solutions. De Wet explores these issues thoroughly, looking at the social determinants of the spread of the disease as well as the configuration and the nature of the responses to it, and their increasing marginalization as factors to address in an era of increased biomedicalization and concomitant normalization.

This book will intrigue scholars and students of public health, global health care, medical sociology, and African Studies.

Katinka de Wet is a Senior Lecturer at the Sociology Department, University of the Free State, South Africa.

Routledge Studies in Health in Africa

Series Editor: Pieter Fourie

The Normalization of the HIV and AIDS Epidemic in South Africa

Katinka de Wet

The Normalization of the HIV and AIDS Epidemic in South Africa

Katinka de Wet

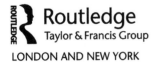

LONDON AND NEW YORK

First published 2020 by Routledge

2 Park Square, Milton Park, Abingdon, Oxon, OX14 4RN
605 Third Avenue, New York, NY 10017

Routledge is an imprint of the Taylor & Francis Group, an informa business

First issued in paperback 2020

British Library Cataloguing-in-Publication Data
A catalogue record for this book is available from the British Library

Library of Congress Cataloging-in-Publication Data
A catalog record has been requested for this book

ISBN: 978-0-367-19355-3 (hbk)
ISBN: 978-0-367-78406-5 (pbk)

Typeset in Bembo
by codeMantra

To the steadfast devotion, patience, and humor of my family, Morné, Roy, and Oliver, words can do no justice.

This book is dedicated to them and to my parents, Zelma, and Jan de Wet

Contents

Acknowledgments

The writing of this book would not have been possible without the support and encouragement from a variety of people. First, I would like to thank my colleagues from the Department of Sociology at the University of the Free State for their interest and assistance all along this journey. In particular, I would like to thank Sethulego Matebesi for being a constant source of encouragement and assistance. The coordinators of the Prestige Scholars Program at the University of the Free State, Professors Jonathan Jansen, Neil Roos, and Jackie du Toit, were instrumental in their conviction that this book project could become a reality. A great word of appreciation goes to our librarians, Lee Goliath, Malefu Mophosho and Jonas Mogopodi. Thanks too, for the intellectual support and "article sharing" from my dear friend Ewa Glapka. Professor Dingie van Rensburg provided me with valued and insightful comments on some of the chapters. His wisdom has always been inspiring. I am also indebted to the editor of the book series Pieter Fourie, for the kind and professional manner in which he dealt with the process from its inception. I benefited from some informal conversations with people from the Treatment Action Campaign and Section 27. I would like to thank, in particular, Loti Rutter and John Stephens. Discussions with Mary Crewe also greatly assisted with some of the ideas that mulled in my mind. Other friends and students who provided moral and intellectual support are Abraham Joubert, Mosilo Machere, Veronica Masenya, Busisiwe Ntsele, Nada Laurie, Jano Coetzee, Lindie Coetzee, Marguerite Muller, Frans Kruger, Gert Hanekom, Laura Drennan, Jane Breet, Wayne Breet, and Lee Murray. The sacrifices and love from my parents continue to make my absence bearable, not only for my two young boys but also for me.

Introduction

The emergence and spread of HIV and AIDS globally has given rise to an abundance of exceptionalities which enabled the AIDS acronym to be thrust into the vocabulary of the banal. HIV and AIDS has attracted unprecedented enquiry (Patton, 2002) inasmuch as its emergence and ramifications have resulted in some of the most extraordinary humanitarian actions in the face of an epidemic (Burchardt, 2014). AIDS was the first health-related topic that was discussed at the UN Security Council in January 2000 as it was pointed out that "AIDS in Africa" constituted a human security crisis (UNAIDS, 2008). For a variety of reasons that will be developed and analyzed in the ensuing pages, HIV has been labeled a "signal pandemic of the global here and now" which, in unprecedented ways, has "exacerbated existing economic and moral divides on an ever more planetary scale" (Comaroff, 2007). The epidemic's ubiquity and fame quickly led to the emergence and proliferation of accounts which explained the "making social of disease" (Frankenberg, 1986). AIDS in the world has become a signifier of many realities, both locally and globally, and through the production of wide-ranging actions spanning from politics, art, and research continues to highlight and expose complex global, structural, and interpersonal entanglements that no other illness succeeded in doing with comparable poignancy, virulence, and sustainability. Although a myriad of similarities to other diseases are shared, HIV and AIDS in its contextual configuration has given rise to what is now widely known as the "AIDS industry." This ubiquitous term, first coined by Cindy Patton (2002), has now come to take on a variety of meanings. In a 2009 special edition of the journal *Social Theory & Health* dedicated to HIV and AIDS in its third decade, Judy Auerbach (in Mykhalovskiy & Rosengarten 2009b) defines the AIDS industry as being

> … a complex system of organizations from multiple sectors, including academia, government, philanthropy, media, industry, and civil society – with institutionalized ways of doing things (from conferences to activism) and funding streams. The goal of the AIDS effort fundamentally is to eradicate AIDS, but it has become difficult to imagine how the complex system that has built up around it will go away should that ever actually occur.
>
> (Mykhalovskiy & Rosengarten, 2009b)

In the editorial of this special edition, the authors also provide a definition of the AIDS industry, adding some additional features to the definition not present in the first rendition. For them, the AIDS industry encapsulates,

> that complex of aid agencies, medical relief organizations, international organizations, NGOs, religious groups, philanthropic organizations, research institutes, an all manner of consultants concerned with HIV as a health crisis of the *"developing" world* – by highlighting new questions about the balance of *prevention and treatment in responding to HIV epidemics in low-income countries* and by furthering pressures *for applied, outcomes-based research*.
>
> (Mykhalovskiy & Rosengarten, 2009a, emphasis added)

This above-mentioned definition also makes mention of the fact that the focus is very much on *where* interventions should be directed at, whereas less attention is paid to whether or not interventions *actually work* (Mykhalovskiy & Rosengarten, 2009a).

An element of suspicion in light of the rise and untamed spread of the AIDS industry is increasingly underscored. This is especially evident in the problematic entanglements of vested interests and AIDS exceptionality. In a study of HIV and AIDS in India, Lawrence Cohen (2005) describes the "politics of competing interests and ideologies" that the AIDS industry often brings about, referring rather to "AIDS cosmopolitanism" which he described as "an imagined formation of dislocated agents using the economically fortified social enterprises of AIDS prevention to support its own covert projects" (Cohen, 2005). Vinh-Kim Nguyen (2004) also redefines the AIDS industry by underscoring its materialization within a postcolonial, free trade context. He calls this industry a "biopolitical assemblage" and indicates that it is "cobbled together from global flows of organisms, drugs, discourses, and technologies of all kinds." Nguyen (2004) suggests that

> as AIDS emerges as the foremost issue threatening economic and political futures in many countries around the world, this AIDS industry has become ever-more entangled with the development industry, a salient example of how humanitarian issues are quietly reconfiguring the contours of Bretton-Woods modernity.

Within the AIDS industry, as in the definition of other social ills that befall our globe at an alarming rate, we see the manifestation of "'open-source anarchy' around global health problems," which Joao Biehl and Adriana Petryna (2013) define as "a policy space in which new strategies, rules, distributive schemes, and the practical ethics of healthcare are being assembled, experimented with, and improvised by a wide array of deeply unequal stakeholders" (Biehl & Petryna, 2013). This is also indicative of the sovereign powers that some of these stakeholders have access to and which allows them to decide on issues of life and death in the face of epidemics but also in light of other disasters, such as displacement, forced migration, famine, and occurrences of natural disasters – in short, all those conditions that strike most flagrantly at those with the least resources to counter these devastations. Catastrophically, AIDS' stronghold is also most secure in low-income countries or among groups whose lives are already characterized by immense forms of precariousness. The complexities linked to HIV are immense. Approximately 75% of HIV transmissions are sexually related – a feature that challenges intervention and mitigation efforts, given the complexity to broach sex and sexuality in an open, nonjudgmental, and frank manner. This has inevitably complicated responses to the epidemic and has led to innumerable challenges within well-intentioned prevention programs. Another feature, more tragic and ironic, is the fact that AIDS decimates especially young adults who have a wide range of familial and financial responsibilities, and these deaths result in infinite consequences for entire families and communities.

Another unprecedented feature of HIV and AIDS that was discernable from the onset manifested in the unusual cooperation and synergy between the epidemic, activism, and science. This feature was precociously identified in the seminal work of Steven Epstein in his book titled *Impure Science. AIDS, Activism, and the Politics of Knowledge* (Epstein, 1996). The AIDS movement is seen as "one of the most astonishing events in the history of global health" (Farmer et al., 2013), and it is therefore unsurprising that there have always been huge stakes at play in the emergence and consequent framing of the disease most studied in humankind. The UN agencies first tasked to deal with this new scourge's ramifications competed fiercely as to ownership of the AIDS agenda as the realization dawned of the proverbial "pot of gold" that this disease held both in terms of potential funding and in terms of its envisaged longevity (Knight, 2006).

However, today, we increasingly witness a growing critique as to the interests and motives of those of us who find ourselves cozily ensconced in this AIDS industry (Chin, 2006; Pisani, 2008) which has to some degree, interesting parallels to a form of "disaster capitalism" (Klein, 2007; Loewenstein, 2016) or "philantro-capitalism" (McGoey, 2015). The central thesis of Naomi Klein's 2007 influential work titled *The Shock Industry. The Rise of Disaster Capitalism* focuses on a critique on the conservative, libertarian economist, Milton Friedman's notion that

> [...] only a crisis – actual or perceived – produces real change. When that crisis occurs, the actions that are taken depend on the ideas that are lying around. That, I believe, is our basic function: to develop alternatives to existing policies, to keep them alive and available until the politically impossible becomes politically inevitable.
>
> (Friedman, 1962 in Klein, 2007)

Klein calls this framing of crisis as "democracy-free-zones" and the above-mentioned theory of Friedman's she names "the shock doctrine." She argues that these "moments of crisis" provide and legitimate decision making that often obscure vested interests and agendas of power and that this happens under the banner of "crisis." In the case of HIV and AIDS, I will argue that the "register of exceptionality" could be understood in a similar manner, given the unprecedented nature of this disease and the uncharacteristic responses it gave rise to.

The concept of "exceptionalism," as initially developed by Walter Benjamin, Carl Schmitt, and taken up extensively by Giorgio Agamben, has been extensively developed to make sense of the hugely discrepant loss of life and unequal politics of treatment that marked and continue to mark to a large extent HIV and AIDS. Schmitt indicates that "the exception is more interesting than the regular case. The rule proves nothing, the exception proves everything" (Schmitt, 1985 in de la Durantaye, 2005). Schmitt's conceptualization revolves around the issue of "sovereignty," which, according to him, is seen as the capacity to decide on the state of exception, and that "the production of the biopolitical body" that can be killed with impunity is "the original activity of sovereign power" (Agamben, 1998). Agamben (1998) also indicates that "a theory of the state of exception is the preliminary condition for any definition of the relation that binds, and at the same time, abandons the living being to law." Neoliberal reforms, market fundamentalism, "feasibility clauses" in progressive documents such as the South African Constitution, and trans-global trade agreements (like the TRIPS agreement) are but some examples of statutory and binding impediments that have paved the way for the early and current responses to AIDS and are largely used as "justification" for nonaction or partial action on the part of the "sovereigns" of our current times. Mbembe (2003) states that this conceptualization of sovereignty indicates "the capacity to define who matters and who does not, who is *disposable* and who is not." It equally reminds us of Nikolas Rose's (2007) notion of the "politics of life itself" where this form of politics is "concerned with our growing capacities to control, manage, engineer, reshape, and modulate the very capacity of human beings as living creatures." This despite the fact that we know and witness on a daily basis that the exact opposite of a "politics of life itself" is tragically possible too.

The focus on exceptionalism in light of "sovereignty" should be complemented with another layer of exceptionalization, which somehow counters the renditions strictly focused on macro, structural constraints. Increasingly, there is a focus on notions of "biological citizenship" (Petryna, 2002; Rose & Novas, 2004), or in light of ART in the time of HIV, Nguyen's (2004) conceptualization of "the emergence of new forms of therapeutic citizenship." "Therapeutic citizenship," according to Nguyen, encompasses "claims made on a global social order on the basis of a therapeutic predicament." HIV and AIDS and its exceptional status gave rise to the proliferation of assemblages that are focusing much more on "agency," and the astonishing turn of various forms of activism that flourished after the emergence of the disease, moving beyond the confines of the nation-state and into biomedical globalization, transnational activism, and humanitarian logic. Nguyen defines "therapeutic citizenship" – in this case being HIV positive and on ART – as an "essentialized identity" or a "biopolitical citizenship," which is "a system of claims and ethical projects that arise out of the conjunction of techniques used to govern populations and govern individual bodies" (Nguyen, 2004). The widespread call for "wider access to lifesaving treatment by a rather unprecedented advocacy coalition encompassing humanitarian organizations and activists, and engaging with governments, donors, researchers and the pharmaceutical industry" started constituting a "therapeutic economy" consisting of "confessional technologies, self-help strategies, and access to drugs in novel ways" (Nguyen, 2004). Surprisingly, Nguyen (2004) is also of the opinion that the current neoliberal landscape is more prone to respond to these "illness claims" than claims based simply on "poverty, injustice or structural violence." HIV and AIDS managed to generate a host of reaction and emotion as a humanitarian issue and, therefore, upheld an equally consummate global media interest that spawned concrete acts of altruism as a variety of donors started to open their coffers with increased intensity as the epidemic progressed with geopolitical strides. It then so happened that, on the one hand, local organizations within countries hard-hit by the epidemic started transforming their programming to incorporate increasingly HIV and AIDS-focused work. On the other hand, entirely new organizations focusing specifically on the disease arose in a short period of time. This unprecedented proliferating of HIV and AIDS work vied with novel and not-so-novel initiatives to garner some of the spoils of global health and government funding. HIV and AIDS led to a truly bandwagon effect as its appeal was strong for an array of actors ranging from celebrities to ecclesiastics. The South African Centre for HIV and AIDS Networking's directory indicates that organizations providing HIV-related health and social welfare services dramatically increased from a couple of hundred organizations in 2003 when it first started doing these inventories, to more than 12,000 organizations by 2012 (Reynolds, 2014). In an oft-heard phrase or innuendo in the corridors of AIDS work, it was truly a "sexy" topic to work on as it bore a magnitude of potential for a host of actors, be they seasoned, expert academics, devoted health professionals, or destitute people living with HIV and AIDS (PLWHAs).

This book, however, is less concerned with the golden years of HIV and AIDS or when the epidemic enjoyed its zenith in terms of interest, focus, and funding. I will argue that the writing is on the wall for the glory years of HIV and AIDS as a unique, exemplary, and exceptional disease. By making this statement, I do not intend to say that HIV and AIDS is not a problematic epidemic anymore, but rather that global and even local attention has shifted to view HIV and AIDS as a disease like any other and to increasingly define it as one issue within a wide range of issues to be dealt with and with equal intensity. HIV and AIDS work is, therefore, becoming increasingly difficult in a context of growing "AIDS fatigue," of magic bullet solutions and quick fixes and where HIV and AIDS orthodoxy is stronger than ever. Also, it is lamented by academics in this field of research, especially by social scientists, as well as by activists, that AIDS just isn't the hot topic that it used to be. In fact, it was an utterance of a Treatment Action Campaign (TAC) representative during the 7th South African AIDS Conference in 2015 that sparked the interest of this book as she lamented that HIV and AIDS "just isn't sexy anymore." Insightfully, Zachy Achmat, who was the first leader and co-founder of the TAC and a vociferous AIDS activist, already identified the potential issue related to the sustainability of HIV and AIDS interests when asked why he wasn't going to attend the 16th International AIDS Conference in Toronto in 2006. He explained,

> Everybody said to me "why did you not go to Toronto [the 16th Inter-national AIDS conference]?" I said, "Sweetie Dear, there [will] be AIDS conferences for another 100 years and I hope to be around for another 50 of them, not for the conference but for those years" … the epidemic is going to last a long, long time and we have to pace ourselves. The biggest prob-lem we face is how we focus political leadership on AIDS as an emergency and on AIDS as a long-term issue. And to maintain that interest in that.
>
> (Achmat, in Knight, 2006)

HIV and AIDS, its science, and the diverse responses to it are increasingly becoming normalized. This process of normalization takes place when pro-cedures and responses become largely institutionalized, bureaucratized, and standardized, and in the case of HIV and AIDS, this progression to normali-zation or "domestication" happens mainly through the extensive and largely successful medicalization of HIV and AIDS. This medicalization, closely as-sociated with "scientific rationality," has the potential to silence divergent and distracting approaches and opinions about disease. Paula Treichler (1999) indicates as much when she mentions,

> science and medicine have traditions through which discursive and bio-logical epidemics are controlled; therefore it disguises contradictions and irrationality.

In fact, through the myriad ethnographic accounts by social and cultural scientists, we know that the current normalized discourses are greatly dis-cordant with many people's real life experiences where HIV intersects with so many other pressing needs, deficiencies, and glaring inequalities.

These inevitable processes of medicalization and rationalization linked to the modern project of attaining global standards to draw accurate comparisons have been well documented elsewhere and point to the triumph of universality over individual complexities in responding to health needs and requirements (Lakoff, 2005; Crane, 2013). But, as Max Weber presciently showed, this process of normalization through institutionalization and bureaucratization has the potential to remove the critical edge of contemplating and reacting toward a newly entrenched status quo. The process of normalization brings with it a strong dose of legitimacy, for without this authority, normalization would normally not occur in the first place. As HIV and AIDS becomes progressively medicalized and normalized, and accepted as such, it becomes increasingly problematic to legitimately criticize the state of affairs. Peter Piot, who was the first executive director of UNAIDS, warned that it would be an enormous error to equate the reasonable need for what he termed "medical normalization" with a "normalization" or "medicalization" of the reaction to HIV and AIDS and thereby abandoning "the need for an exceptional response in terms of specific leadership, financing and policies" (Piot in Knight, 2006).

Also, the AIDS apocalypse, as was once predicted or rather prophesized, never took place, which also subsided many of the initial fears and anxieties that were imminent during the so-called "plague years." Much-improved data started indicating that the epidemic was actually starting to stabilize in terms of prevalence, and this happened at the same time as the expanded international response was at its peak. The predictions of complete anarchy and state collapse in southern and eastern African areas, which were labeled the "epicenter" of the disease and where prevalence was shown to be increasingly problematic, also did not happen. The predicted "break out" from concentrated to generalized epidemics in so-called "second wave" countries (like China, India, Russia, Eastern European countries, Central Asia, South and South-East Asia) never ensued (Ingram, 2013). In fact, the "end of AIDS?" was – at a very early stage – already imagined with a headline of a 1996 *Newsweek* cover story after the groundbreaking discovery of highly active antiretroviral therapy or HAART (in Crane, 2013).

This initial euphoria was quickly tempered by the alarming reports of AIDS' devastating consequences in Africa and the alarmist predictions that followed in its wake. But the first world and third world realities continued to be separated with the emergence of various terms that signaled the demise of a former AIDS era. Kane Race indicates a new vocabulary that came to characterize the dawn of HAART (Race, 2001). As early as 1996, Gary Dowsett and David McInnes, for example, coined the term "post-AIDS" to indicate the diminished sense of AIDS being "experienced as a communal crisis" among Australian gay men (Dowsett & McInnes, 1996, in Race, 2001). As for the USA, Eric Rofes adopted a similar term to describe the experiences of gay men in the USA. He describes the aftermath of the HAART announcement in 1996 at the International AIDS Conference in Vancouver, Canada, in the following terms,

> All social and cultural changes in our experiences of the AIDS epidemic were explained in light of the new therapies, or "the cocktail" as "the Protease Moment."
>
> (Rofes, 1998, in Race, 2001)

The dream, so long deferred by pricing and politics of generalized access to antiretroviral therapy (ART) in the rest of the world – notably in the global South – where the treatment was most needed, only slowly started to become a reality in the early 2000s. The immense success of global ART access that led to significantly prolonging PLWHA's lives has been nothing less than astounding and has even led to suggesting the "decoupling" of HIV from AIDS in this post-ART era (Rosengarten, 2010), thereby denoting the widening gap between HIV as a chronic, manageable condition, on the one hand, and AIDS as a death sentence, on the other. However, Rosengarten (2009) equally calls ART an "unsatisfactory privilege" to convey her view that ART in itself is not a satisfactory intervention to address HIV nor the disease in its duality (HIV *and* AIDS), for that matter. As critical scholars will concur, a solely biomedical response will never do justice to an epidemic as vast and as complex as HIV, and even if an effective vaccine has to be put to use immediately, AIDS consequences and AIDS assemblages are firmly entrenched in global health configurations. Moreover, many people still die of AIDS, children are still born with HIV infection, and prevention still fails to thwart new infections. The "pharmaceuticalization" of HIV (Biehl, 2007) has been accused of separating patient care from other issues such as nutrition, mental health, housing, stigmatization, and poverty and social justice in general. Also, in the process of medicalization or pharmaceuticalization, those on treatment who fail to comply or to adhere according to the prescribed regimes are merely branded as "non-compliant" or "poorly adherent," thereby completely discounting the context in which these people find themselves – a situation often characterized by extreme forms of marginalization and precariousness.

In light of HIV and AIDS' dwindling legitimacy as "exceptional": perceived, real, or disputed, and its concurrent overwhelming "biomedical focus," this book will aim to convey another look at the "end of AIDS." This rendition is steeped in Francis Fukayama's original thesis which appeared more than 25 years ago. His thesis developed in *The End of History* predicts that liberal democracy as witnessed in some parts of the developed world, in effect means an end to humanity's sociocultural evolution as this will always be the form of government that will be striven toward or adhered to. There is a striking similarity between Fukayama's idea of the "end of history" – or the notion that we have reached a level of perfection that will always be striven toward (liberal democracy) – and the HIV and AIDS treatment successes (the widespread availability of live-saving ART after the "dying years" of AIDS). This similarity is especially apparent in the manner in which ART has manifested in the South African context where a unique history of HIV and AIDS has led to reconfiguring and reimagining novel notions related to civil rights and citizenship, and where new forms of "biosociality" (Rabinow, 1996) are forged in this post-ART era. So, the aforementioned "liberal democracy" in Fukayama's account could be substituted by the gamut of chemical treatments (ART) available to those infected with HIV in the South African context. But over the years, Fukayama reviewed his original thesis, although still strongly adherent to this initial idea,

> The biggest single problem in societies aspiring to be democratic has been their failure to provide the substance of what people want from government: personal security, shared economic growth and the basic public services (especially education, health care and infrastructure) that are needed to achieve individual opportunity. Proponents of democracy focus, for understandable reasons, on limiting the powers of tyrannical or predatory states. But they don't spend as much time thinking about how to govern effectively. They are, in Woodrow Wilson's phrase, more interested in "controlling than in energizing government."
>
> (Fukayama, 2014)

Fukayama's revision of his theory is interesting if the parallel is to be taken further. In the context of HIV, ART's hegemony (like that of liberal democracy) is globally secure as the biomedical status quo grows in stature and status because of its immense potential to guarantee survival. However, this guarantee of life might be conditional as it depends on ongoing global health funding; it often creates new inequalities as some system of triage – globally and locally – still applies and as access and the quality of medication differ between the global South and North. ART and other biomedical interventions might guarantee life but not necessarily quality of life; it might give rise to collateral damage because of perverse vested interests of politicians, corporations, academics, and scientists; it might provide the promise of survival but at the expense of deeper structural transformations that have the potential to lead to more sustainable solutions rooted in global social justice; it might warrant continued existence, but often targets and statistics drive the thrust to get people onto treatment at the expense of quality and mindful interventions. As with liberal democracy and the promises it holds for our globe, the seemingly panacea of ART should also be continually questioned and scrutinized and certainly not be taken for granted.

Imagine what would have been lost in the analysis of HIV and AIDS in South Africa if the epidemic was not used as a mirror reflecting the complex history of the South African society? The story of HIV and AIDS is that of South Africa's history, as it exposes the fragility of this democracy by unearthing persistent inequalities on multiple levels. Post-AIDS or the "end of AIDS" in the context of South Africa, the epicenter of the disease with more than seven million people infected (Republic of South Africa, 2017) is equally revealing of an array of realities at both a macro and a micro level, and the disease has taken unexpected turns in the past couple of decades. The incredulity as to the biomedical inroads that the country has made was often reiterated during the 7th South African AIDS Conference held in June 2015 by people who have a good track record of combining science and activism. In the words of Dr Francois Venter, well-known medical practitioner in both scientific and activist circles of the South African HIV and AIDS milieu, our biomedical strides in terms of ART access were "unthinkable" a mere 10 years ago. But these advances are shadowed by ever-emerging new realities as to the daily negotiation of HIV and even of AIDS in terms of living with the disease, having access to medications, providing care for those with HIV and AIDS, sustaining activism in light of the scourge, and rethinking the research landscape that is rapidly changing not only because of financial restrictions but also because of HIV and AIDS losing its unique standing in the global health picture. HIV and AIDS – coupled and decoupled – continues to mark an unabated state of complexity which is constantly in flux and which re-quires an ongoing re-reconfiguring of the disease that is still wreaking havoc despite the intense onslaught of a biomedical colonization. Noises are also made that continued and expanded roll-out of ART is not sustainable and that, according to a South African expert, we cannot "treat our way out of this epidemic" (Fourie & Swart, 2014). This statement obviously flies in the face of the direction taken by the South African Ministry of Health, which unequivocally and without deliberations with the South African National AIDS Council (SANAC), was the first African country to accept the UN-AIDS' biomedical 90:90:90 initiative with the vision of leading South Africa to an AIDS-free generation in 2030.[1]

The word "nostalgia" is increasingly used to refer back to the "good old bad days of AIDS," albeit in different contexts and registers. This sense of nostalgia is felt and expressed under a wide-ranging rubric, probably most famously articulated by the recent "clash" between "old" and "new" gen-eration HIV-positive gay men in the USA with the much debated art work titled "Your Nostalgia is killing me" (Visual AIDS, 2014), imploring the older generation to make way for a new voice in AIDS advocacy circles. The stronghold of the older generation, firmly rooted in their immense impact in the early years of AIDS in the USA of an organization such as Act Up[2] is thus being challenged and is indicative of emerging tensions between "AIDS generations" all over the world as we find ourselves in the fourth decade of dealing with HIV and AIDS. Also, in her work on the development of HIV and AIDS work in Uganda, Crane (2013) juxtaposes the "old," romanticized, qualitative manner in which HIV and AIDS was treated by doctors – using a good dose of humanity, care, and clinical estimation to treat the disease compared to the "new," molecularized, standardized, technocratized way that has almost entirely engulfed the sentient touch of the early days of HIV and AIDS care. Relebohile Moletsane's AIDS Review with the simple title *Nostalgia* also analyzes this issue but does so in a much more forward-looking manner by questioning and analyzing the representations of HIV and AIDS that have been created and forged over the years (Moletsane, 2014). The tense and increasingly scrutinized ethics in relations between the "North" and the "South," and even between "equals in the South," in the face of HIV and AIDS research is assessed and reflected upon. As for a potential meaning of nostalgia, she quotes Jill Broadbent who suggests that

Perhaps nostalgia is not so much a longing for the way things were, as a longing for futures that never came or horizons of possibility that have been foreclosed by the unfolding of events. Perhaps nostalgia is the desire not to be who we once were but to be once again our potential selves.

(Broadbent, in Moletsane, 2014)

In its biomedical, bureaucratized, and molecularized wake, the AIDS industry, as we know it (and which we might reminisce about), becomes increasingly endangered. I will set out to paint this picture, first by describing how HIV and AIDS acquired its unique and exceptional status since the early 1990s. Its "exceptional" status is inscribed under a host of registers, a list that I will expand upon that normally informs the "exceptionality" debate, and Chapter 1 outlines these various registers to demonstrate how HIV and AIDS was and continues to be framed differently from other diseases. This chapter demonstrates that the exceptional manner in which HIV and AIDS has been depicted since it first emerged as a disease, serves as a heuristic analytical grid to trace interactions between global and local discourses of HIV and AIDS.

Chapter 2 situates South Africa within the context of "global health" by tracing the meaning and origins of this relatively new term and by situating HIV and AIDS and its lifesaving treatment within its mandate. This chapter argues that, despite South Africa's large investments in its own HIV and AIDS programs, we are still heavily reliant upon foreign aid and outside largess. It also shows how the money dedicated to the South African program largely goes toward biomedical interventions at the expense of other, notably social funding objectives.

As this book is about crises of legitimacy of an exceptional disease at various levels, it will also set out to show how formerly applauded initiatives pale into insignificance and even disregard in the post-AIDS era. In Chapter 3, the role and history of the newly formed cadre of "Community Health Workers" is described and juxtaposed with the 2014 retrenchment of over 3,000 such workers in the Free State Province (South Africa) and ensuing court action against some of these destitute workers who marched onto the provincial Department of Health as a form of protest against this decision. The emergence of Community Health Workers was a highly praised initiative that gained tremendous ground during the period that marked the peak of AIDS deaths before the advent of ART (an era in which they mostly rendered so-called home-based care). Today, this group also fulfills a significant role in the phase of generalized access to this lifesaving treatment and guidelines as to primary healthcare reengineering, and the notion of "task-shifting" embrace this new cadre as part of the healthcare system following hugely successful examples of such initiatives in other under-resourced areas with high morbidity prevalence. However, the Free State example shows that this lay-initiative, a test of alternative claims to citizenship (reminiscent of the conceptualization of "biological citizenship" or "therapeutic citizenship") with strong connotations to HIV and AIDS, is not resilient to haphazard politicking given its contested and undefined status in the country despite its existence for well over a decade.

Another sustainable enterprise that increasingly sees its funding cut has been the HIV and AIDS activist domain within South Africa – a phenomenon that has also been witnessed globally. With the advent of treatment that ironically came about because of unparalleled activism, HIV activists in South Africa have had to reinvent themselves to guarantee their legitimacy in the face of decreased funding and a dwindling interest in the disease. Chapter 4 looks at this decline in activism's legitimacy and describes the ways in which activism has reinvented itself in order to respond to the changing landscape of post-AIDS and all the realities that accompany this shift in focus. Although not in the limelight anymore, South Africa's activism in the form of the well-known organization, the Treatment Action Campaign (TAC), and organizations such as Section 27 are fulfilling an important role in this purported unproblematic era of biomedicalization by continuing to occupy an "uncomfortable space"[3] that few dare to enter in a seemingly successful context of ART roll-out, access, and successes.

The final chapter, Chapter 5, is set on contemplating the future of HIV and AIDS as a topic of research, especially among social and cultural scientists, as it is within this field that the crisis of legitimacy is most acutely experienced. I argue that those of us in the AIDS industry will have to reinvent the ways in which we conceive of research by taking into consideration the constant transformation of ethics related to HIV and AIDS research, and by seriously questioning the relevance of our research in this constantly changing landscape.

These chapters, seemingly disparate, adhere to Nguyen's (2004) observation related to the extraordinary manner in which HIV and AIDS has brought together such altogether distinct occurrences "into a remarkably stable, worldwide formation," or "assemblages" which again posits a level of exceptionalism that marks this epidemic. This book is also unashamedly about South Africa, where the world's greatest amount of HIV-positive people live and where the largest ART program ever to exist, is growing daily. There is a fine balance, in writing yet another book on HIV and AIDS, not to do so just for the sake of it. Moreover, writing a social scientific rendition of HIV and AIDS could easily be considered to fall into what has been described as the "Luddite trap." The Luddites were a group of textile workers who, in the 19th-century England, destroyed textile machines as an act of revolt as they saw in these machines the substitution of their unique skills in the textile industry. This appellation, therefore, became equivalent to any kind of reservation or critique against technology. In this monograph's case, it might seem as if biomedical strides and inroads are being criticized unreasonably. The reckoning might be that people now access (on an ever-growing scale) treatment for HIV, that HIV has become manageable and a chronic condition, and that this treatment is becoming all the more efficacious and sophisticated. So why still the necessity to "denounce" these rightfully successful interventions? First, technological advances in medicine might bring about new hope for prolonging biological life, but biological life is sometimes devoid of social, economic, or political life. These forms of life might be so precarious that the hope of biological life is not that promising after all. Paul Farmer (1999) indicates as much when he notes that "effacing the inequality of outcomes is not the same as eliminating the underlying forces of inequality itself." Second, social inequalities do not only shape the manner in which epidemics emerge all over the world but also determine the health outcomes of those who are afflicted by epidemics or other social ills. And third, by tracing the historical roots of the manner in which other diseases have been responded to, it is rather unsettling to imagine that a similar fate might await the HIV and AIDS epidemic. Slow, bureaucratic mechanisms and organizations that dictate the direction and the intensity of responses are to be held to intense scrutiny by accountable and ethical global actors in order to deflect a destiny for HIV that is similar to an epidemic such as tuberculosis (TB). This book is, therefore, a contribution to the existing critique of processes of biomedicalization and normalization not to discredit these lifesaving endeavors but rather to understand the myriad pitfalls and challenges that these processes potentially and concretely harbor. It will try to understand the manner in which history continues to repeat itself, where AIDS is a reflection of responses that characterize a wide variety of disease manifestations and other humanitarian disasters, perpetuating the "dialectic of history and power, capital and geopolitics" (Comaroff, 2010).

Notes

1 The 90:90:90 targets are set to be achieved by 2020, and projects to have 90% of the world's population living with HIV, to know their status. The second 90% refers to the projection that by 2020, 90% of all people who have been diagnosed with HIV will be receiving continual antiretroviral therapy (ART); whereas the last 90% refers to the expectation that 90% of all people who receive this ART will be viral suppressant (UNAIDS, 2014).
2 The AIDS Coalition to Unleash Power (Act Up) is a US-based civil organization that saw the day after AIDS started killing gay men in the USA and as a result of political apathy and inaction to respond to this tragedy. It was created in 1987 at the Lesbian and Gay Services Centre in New York and mustered an impressive amount of expertise combined with civil activism to change the course of HIV history as it was written globally.
3 Dr Francois Venter made this reference to the TAC during a comment when he was the facilitator at a plenary session of the 7th South African AIDS Conference in 2015.

1 From exceptionality to ordinariness

How HIV and AIDS lost its sex appeal

HIV and AIDS' rise to prominence is rooted in its exceptional manifestation in a global context that was conducive to this unique historical trajectory. This exceptionality takes on an even more dramatic form in the contemporary South African environment most obviously because of the fact that South Africa has the greatest amount of HIV-positive people globally and that it boasts the greatest antiretroviral therapy (ART) program on the planet. South Africa also tragically witnessed the rise of HIV and AIDS among its citizens shortly after the victory that marked the prolonged fight against the injustices of apartheid. This is reminiscent of the uncanny forewarning made by Chris Hani[1] in 1990, when he uttered, "We cannot afford to allow the AIDS epidemic to ruin the realization of our dreams" (in Fassin, 2007).

The "exceptionality debate" is a useful analytical instrument to trace the flux of discourses related to the HIV and AIDS scourge, globally but also locally. South Africa's responses, greatly shaped and defined by unprecedented activism for ART access, were initially influenced by global – especially American – HIV activism triggered in the early 1980s. Today, this exceptional status is under threat for a variety of reasons, but chiefly because of the normalization through biomedicalization being at the root of rendering HIV and AIDS like any other disease. HIV and AIDS as a unique and exceptional disease is losing its erstwhile appeal, and it seems as if the "glory days" of HIV and AIDS might be transferred to the annals of its exclusive and spectacular history. It is also rather worrisome to see the once vibrant, socially conscious AIDS movements' prominence dwindling in a climate of neoliberalism marked by increasing competition, austerity, and scarcity. In fact, this state of affairs could increasingly be linked to the notion of a "politics of abandonment" (Ingram, 2013), especially in light of other pressing matters also clambering for attention and in a situation where former attractiveness and allure of the HIV disease is just not that robust anymore.

The devastating and ubiquitous HIV and AIDS epidemic has been around "officially"[2] for more than three decades and, in its wake, has left many global citizens dead, doomed, destitute, or depressed. The epidemic has taken on surprising epidemiological turns which till this day baffle ordinary people and experts alike. From a disease concentrated among homosexual, affluent communities in mostly Western countries, it manifested disproportionately in some parts of the developing world, especially in sub-Saharan Africa where it reached staggering levels of prevalence especially among heterosexual, "black" African people. For years, an arsenal of visual representations appeared to portray emaciated and diseased bodies: images directly linked to the slow, excruciating, and undignified way in which people lived and died with AIDS. Before the availability of highly active antiretroviral therapy (HAART) that first became obtainable in 1996 – but at exorbitant and largely unattainable prices for the majority of those afflicted by AIDS – death because of AIDS was more equally distributed as ultimate progression to full-blown AIDS inevitably led to a person's demise. The premature deaths of prominent, affluent figures such as Michel Foucault, Freddie Mercury, and Rock Hudson evidenced this equalizing force of a disease without treatment. More easily forgotten though are the millions of faceless fatalities due to AIDS even after HAART became available.

Much has been studied, reported, debated, and disputed within the realm of the HIV and AIDS empire. In fact, staggering amounts of resources have gone into and are still earmarked for HIV and AIDS research. In the current context of normalization, this especially encompasses efforts to mitigate the impact of the epidemic which translate into biomedical treatment programs. Biomedical research in the form of randomized controlled trials in view of improved treatment or an eventual vaccine or even a cure are commonplace. Studies in the social sciences and humanities are equally well represented, and dedicated journals, research institutes, literature, films, and global activist groupings all strive to offer alternative views of a disease that signifies much more than a mere biomedical manifestation within bodies. The genealogy of "discourses" of HIV and AIDS has been studied from various points of view. This chapter will equally trace the origins and sequels that reflect some HIV and AIDS discourses that act as *definitions of an illness* within a particular context. These definitions, in turn, ultimately determine the construction of *responses* aimed toward addressing this affliction (De Cock et al., 2002).

HIV and AIDS is an epidemic with manifold ramifications, more so than other similar (and deadly) diseases, and this uniqueness has given rise to the widely used term "HIV exceptionalism." Its exceptional character is complex and manifold, and this "exceptionality" will be the background against which to pose this monograph's chapters. Contextualizing the phenomenon called AIDS exceptionalism also needs to be understood as emerging in a global climate that is marked by a host of global realities. One such contextual reality was the post-Cold War environment that prepared a fertile ground for the AIDS epidemic to become exceptional. This period, marked by narratives of injustice and crime, "reparation politics," and revisionist histories characterized by a "memory boom," is indicative of this global climate. Olick (2007) indicates the "increase in redress claims, the rise of identity politics, a politics of victimisation and regret, and an increase willingness of governments to acknowledge wrongdoing." This was "all part of the decline of the memory-nation as an unchallengeable hegemonic force" (Olick, 2007). The ethical values in the post-Cold War context, therefore, changed considerably. International relations were viewed as being "conflict prone and anarchic" during the Cold War years, and there was a generalized view that no central authority could control states' actions. In this context, states were acting to maximize the realization of their own material interests. However, the post-Cold War years were increasingly influenced by the important role that non-state actors could play to change the norms of entire states and to affect their interests (Mbali, 2013).

In fact, rights issues stood central at the onset of the AIDS epidemic as it arrived shortly after the sexual revolution as well as the feminist, gay rights, and patients' rights movements. The AIDS epidemic was seen as a major test of political commitment (Scheper-Hughes, 1994). Scheper-Hughes (1994) indicates that the exceptionality of the AIDS epidemic was made possible because of its initial framing as a crisis in human rights (with obvious public health ramifications) "rather than a crisis in public health that had some important human rights dimensions." The novelty of this focus – on rights and not on the disease *per se* – disregarded and largely reconfigured classic responses of public health. The substitution of responses characterized by collective, obligatory, and, at times, invasive measures by an approach focused more on "education and voluntarism," crafted the responses of the early AIDS years (Scheper-Hughes, 1994).

In addition, the 1960s and 1970s saw an alarming increase in the "medicalization" of many aspects of life. An expanding index of ordinary life events were being framed as "diseases" requiring technological and biomedical interventions (Nguyen, 2010). According to Nguyen (2010),

> As Europe and North America were swept by a diverse array of counter-cultural movements with roots in the American civil-rights movement in the late 1960s, a robust resistance to medicalisation emerged […]. Therefore, the notions of community development and patient empowerment that AIDS activism advocated emerged from the social environment that existed when the epidemic appeared in the major cities of North America in 1981.

This unique confluence of global events greatly paved the way for the exceptional unfolding of a unique disease. By "exceptional," I mean that a "business-as-usual" approach to addressing the epidemic was not harnessed, as was witnessed from the early 1980s when AIDS started to wreak havoc among homosexual men in the United States of America (USA). The unexpected occurrence of this infectious disease led to widespread public fear and panic as homosexual men started dying in great numbers. In addition, this rise in infections and death saw an unprecedented effort by these mostly homosexual activists to campaign for a "civil liberties" approach toward those infected (Smith & Whiteside, 2010). This strong lobby succeeded in largely abandoning conventional public health procedures like universal screening, routine testing, partner notification, quarantine, and other classic epidemic control measures (Nguyen & Sama, 2008). It rather paved the way toward a "rights-based" or a "civil liberties" approach to HIV infection and AIDS, by notably stressing individual choice in testing and disclosure. This should be understood as first happening in a time of immense uncertainty as there was no treatment available to manage HIV infection and AIDS. Despite many subsequent changes to this approach, it has been argued that the "rights-based" approach that was subsequently transplanted in Africa from the early HIV years in the USA was not necessarily a good match for the manner in which the epidemic manifested in this part of the world. In fact, one author equates this "rights-based" approach, that has led to differentiating HIV and AIDS from other infectious diseases and its concomitant heightened stigmatization, to the promotion of an "African holocaust" (Alcorn, 2001 in Nguyen & Sama, 2008).

Smith and Whiteside's (2010) article on the history of AIDS exceptionalism is an authoritative elucidation of the genesis of this terminology. The term "HIV exceptionalism" first appeared in 1991 in an article in the *New England Journal of Medicine*. Interestingly, the very debates around the term "exceptionalism" were starting to "transform into the subject of controversy" (Oppenheimer & Bayer, 2009). Whereas this term originally designated largely compatible policy results, it soon surfaced as a site for contestation. Especially related to testing (i.e. HIV testing being differentiated in terms of requiring informed consent, or pre- and post-counseling), more stakeholders started seeing this facet of exceptionalism as posing a barrier to transforming HIV from a clinical and public health point of view. Those more in favor of the "new rights-protective regime" downplayed the salience of the term "exceptionalism" and rather emphasized the successful configuration of public health practice that emerged after AIDS became a common signifier. This debate, therefore, indicated, soon after AIDS emerged as a powerful signifier, that "any effort to force HIV into a preconceived or traditional mold of public health would be counterproductive" (Oppenheimer & Bayer, 2009).

Framing HIV and AIDS as exceptional has other consequences as well, especially related to the use and procurement of drugs in the early years. Not only was mass testing discouraged, but the emergency and exceptional status of the disease led to the use (at times) of substandard drugs or the procurement of counterfeit products. Activism's insistence on making treatment available at all cost, gave rise to the concept of "cataclysmic rights" – thereby fast-tracking drugs, like the use of AZT in the early days of HIV, to respond to the dramatic character of AIDS and its immediate aftermath. Trials did not run their full duration and were referred to as "compassionate release trials" to afford people a glimmer of hope in the devastating prospects brought about by AIDS (see Patton, 1990b). This has also been referred to as "politics of strategic reductionism" (Comaroff, 2007), which in effect meant that drugs were made available under pressure from activists even if their results and effects were not certain.

Early tensions that erupted between AIDS exceptionalism and the normalization of AIDS have continued unabated. A well-known South African expert of HIV and AIDS, Alan Whiteside calls the arguments between AIDS exceptionalism and the normalization of HIV, "sterile" (Whiteside, 2009). This statement stems largely from the frustration that some researchers, politicians, people living with HIV and AIDS (PLWHAs), and activists experience in light of the unrelenting suffering that this epidemic *and* its consequences still cause in many parts of the globe, especially in sub-Saharan Africa. In fact, Whiteside (2009) indicates that those millennium development goals (MDGs) that have not obtained desired results were all because of the devastating consequences of HIV and AIDS. Therefore, Whiteside argues that HIV exceptionality should rather be framed as being a "developmental issue," as has been indicated by many other stakeholders (Collins & Rau, 2000). As is necessary in these debates, Whiteside (2009) creates a rational explanation – grounded in epidemiology – to motivate the sole reasons why HIV should be considered exceptional. He divides countries into two categories: those with "mid-range prevalence of between 3 and 10%, and those countries with a prevalence of more than 10%." First, for the mid-range prevalence countries, the "exceptionality rule" is a function of "prevalence and wealth" except for most-at-risk populations (MARPs). Whiteside puts it plainly: in places where people can access treatment, AIDS should not be considered exceptional. However, this picture changes where treatment is reliant on outside funding and where PLWHAs are benefitting from higher spending per individual compared to per capita health expenditure in the country as a whole. The reason why HIV and AIDS is still exceptional in these circumstances is related to their dependence on "international largess," and the fact that being HIV-positive (economically) favors HIV-positive people over others who might have equally serious health-related conditions.

As for countries with a prevalence of 10% or more, Whiteside (2009) argues that HIV and AIDS cannot (and should not) be seen in any other light other than being exceptional. Whiteside mentions the huge demographic and social consequences when this level of prevalence is present, especially when left untreated. De Cock et al. (2002) develop another argument where normalization and exceptionality are seen as mere concepts,

> The normalization of HIV/AIDS in a philosophical context of public health, medical ethics, and social justice is not a threat to individual human rights; rather, failure to prevent HIV transmission constitutes an infringement of human rights that hampers Africa's human and social development.

This quote is equally indicative of the level of frustration with this seemingly academic squabbling and philosophizing to the detriment, some would say of concrete, lifesaving action. This critique probably confirms the crux of Whiteside's argument in that the debate between exceptionalism and normalization is unproductive and rather obsolete. In this chapter, I will disagree with the statement that the debate between "exceptionalism" and "normalization" is sterile and obsolete. In fact, this tension avails a heuristic analytical framework to conceptualize the unprecedented occurrence of HIV and AIDS not only in highly affected areas but also in contexts of low prevalence where biopolitics are securely entrenched. A debate that pitches exceptionalism against normalization not only assists in tracing the genealogy of HIV and AIDS as it happened in the so-called "developed" global North with its unprecedented solidarity and activism in the face of HIV but also elucidates the manner in which a country like South Africa's responses were shaped and crafted under the register of exceptionality. In fact, the narratives of exceptionality, notably as they emerged in the USA, can be juxtaposed with the narratives of exceptionality in South Africa, despite the many divergences of the two countries. Moreover, it is interesting to reflect on the manner in which the first responses to AIDS in the developed world shaped the subsequent responses *vis-à-vis* the epidemic in the South African context. Also, it is the construction of exceptionalism that has rendered the study of HIV and AIDS appealing to researchers all over the globe and led to emphasizing those economic and moral divides that mark our world. Notions of "sovereignty," as described in the Introduction (the power to decide over life and death), issues of tragic triage, but also the construction of new forms of claims to citizenship under conditions of precariousness, are all converging rather arbitrarily, to further consolidate the issue of "exceptionalism" in light of HIV and AIDS. Today, as this exceptional status is dwindling and HIV is fashioned as "just another disease," a great deal is at stake for some groupings, including activists, health workers, politicians, entire countries dependent on foreign aid, and those infected and affected by HIV.

Smith and Whiteside (2010) place the exceptionality debate related to the disease into two broad registers. First, they underscore the lethality of the syndrome, which solicited a concomitant urgent response. Second, they identify the unprecedented investment of resources to address the epidemic by international aid and by countries' own contributions as well. In this chapter, I will expand on the notion of exceptionality linked to HIV and AIDS by adding more layers to their insightful classification, thus creating a more encompassing taxonomy of exceptionality. Under some registers, I contrast discourses emanating from the USA with those from South Africa in order to show some continuities between the two contexts. I will also consider the fluctuations of these discourses by including various sources of critique that aim to render HIV more "normalized" or "mainstream" (Oppenheimer & Bayer, 2009) and, therefore, less "exotic."

The rest of this chapter will thus focus on five identified layers of exceptionalism:

1   Etiological exceptionalism,
2   Resources exceptionalism,

3   Rights exceptionalism,
4   Moralistic exceptionalism, and
5   South African exceptionalism.

Etiological exceptionalism

The first point of entry to understand HIV's exceptional character is vested in its specific *disease manifestation*. This specifically refers to its lethality when left untreated, its long, dangerous incubation period in which the vector of HIV can spread the virus unknowingly and imperceptibly[3]; the virulence of its spread; the unexpected nature of its occurrence; its specific gendered and geographical range that assumes staggering expression in sub-Saharan Africa; its exceptional response in terms of treatment; and the many uncertainties about HIV that still lurk in the near future. As early as 1996, a report at the International AIDS Conference in Vancouver explained the immense complexity of the disease, referring to ways the infection has been fragmented, rendering it more apt to refer to "diseases" rather than one single disease (Knight, 2006).

HIV/AIDS as "diseases"

> (…) a uniform global approach might not be suited to the extreme geographical and epidemiological heterogeneity of the pandemic.
>
> (De Cock et al., 2002)

Former South African president Thabo Mbeki believed (and might still believe) that HIV does not cause AIDS, and that the unprecedented number of deaths ascribed to HIV should rather be assigned to the toll of poverty.[4] Peter Piot (2008), who was the first executive director of UNAIDS (1996–2008), and in no way an adherent of AIDS denialism, stated that HIV is not a disease of poverty but rather a disease of *inequality*, and he underscored the fact that gender inequality, or the "feminization of the epidemic," is the starkest example of this injustice (Piot, 2008). In fact, Piot problematizes the wording that refers to HIV as "the global HIV epidemic" and states that this homogenizing language is not an accurate depiction of this epidemic, and that it should rather be understood and explained in its plurality: as *diseases*. Yeboah (2007) aptly calls HIV a "global virus with transcultural implications."

Although Africa is home to only 15% of the global population, it houses 70% of the world's HIV and AIDS infections. This skewed burden of disease is compounded by the fact that Africa as a continent lives on 1% of the global economy (World Health Organization (WHO), 2014). This glaring inequality is also evident in the "80-20 divide" where it was reported in the 2010 Health Expenditure Report that 84% of annual global health spending is earmarked to respond to the needs of 18% of the world's population (Van Niekerk, 2014). In its gendered manifestation, statistics tell us that 75% of those infected in the 17- to 24-year-old category are female (UNAIDS, 2013). It is thus hardly surprising that the experience of HIV is not a homogeneous event as is evident in its unequal epidemiological dispersion but also in growing global inequities when considering the manner in which the global resources pie is divided in order to respond to the burden of disease.

Normalization through biomedicalization

Shortly after stepping down as UNAIDS' first executive director, Peter Piot reflected on the global HIV and AIDS experience. He recalled the historic meeting of the UN General Assembly, a special session on HIV and AIDS, which *the Economist* later branded "the turning point in the global response to AIDS." At this high-level meeting, Piot mentioned that all donors and representatives present at the meeting (Africa and Asia were also represented), with the exception of France, were opposed to commit to any goals or targets related to ART. This meeting, after an "absurd debate all night long," was the first step toward a loose commitment to universal access to treatment (Piot, 2008). The initial arguments hinged on the fact that ART could not be provided to people in the developing world due to the complexities of the ART regimen. It was also widely believed by the representatives that those living in precarious conditions would not be able to comply with treatment, and that health systems in these poor countries would not be able to manage the logistics associated with HIV treatment. However, initial pilot programs initiated by organizations such as *Médecins Sans Frontières* contradicted these initial assumptions and experts started providing evidence related to the benefits of ART. This evidence especially pointed to the fact that the treatment significantly lengthened people's lives, thereby outweighing the potential costs involved in scaling-up treatment. This argument was in line with the prevailing human rights claim that put people's lives first. The WHO announced its "3 × 5" campaign, which aimed toward placing three million people on treatment by 2005. In 2006, 111 countries, of which South Africa was one, committed to achieving universal access[5] to prevention, treatment, care, and support by 2010 (Smith & Whiteside, 2010). This ambitious initiative, therefore, promoted expanded ART access but did not actually provide funding for this treatment. The ambitious target of three million was met, but only two years later in 2007.

Despite the immense successes witnessed in global ART programs, the lives saved and prolonged and sustained efforts to expand on access, the drugs continued to be expensive, and beyond the reach of many of those infected. Furthermore, patients will inevitably have to move from first-line treatment to more costly second-line treatments as resistance will start affecting those who have been on treatment for some time (Whiteside, 2009). The goalposts of treatment eligibility are constantly shifting, and the WHO now advises that people start treatment as soon as possible after diagnosis with HIV infection. The focus is, therefore, not on CD4 counts anymore, as was the case until recently. It has been shown that increased treatment active populations will also lead to better prevention outcomes as those on ART are said to develop lower and even undetectable viral loads or viral suppression (which is responsible for infection), and higher CD4 counts (which are important for a strong immune system, productivity and "normalcy"). In fact, UNAIDS are commercializing and branding this new vision of treatment and its anticipated outcomes as the 90:90:90 ambition.[6]

These ambitious targets, even acknowledged as such by UNAIDS,[7] are set to reach the even more aspiring target of "the end of AIDS in 2030" (UNAIDS, 2014b). In addition, South Africa was the first country to adopt unambiguously the 90:90:90 UNAIDS vision that will purportedly lead to an end of AIDS by 2030. In fact, South Africa has also been the first country in which provision is made in the public sector for third-line regimen treatment to those who have become resistant to other lines of treatment (Maartens, 2015).

The biomedicalization of prevention

Prevention has been approached from various angles since HIV first started manifesting as a generalized public health concern. It is now widely acknowledged that the "ABC" of prevention is, in fact, not that commonsensical after all and that it has proven to be woefully ineffective. "A" for abstain, "B" indicating that lovers should "be faithful," and "C" indicating that sexually active people should use condoms comprised this seemingly simple AIDS alphabet. In fact, many initial globally funded HIV programs were concentrated exclusively on this rudimentary message of prevention at the expense of treatment programs, or for that matter, more insightful prevention programs. Prevention, although always featuring in discourses and omnipresent in the fight against the HIV scourge, has proven difficult to implement, to sustain, and to legitimize. Peter Piot (2008) fittingly describes prevention by stating, "Prevention is about counting non-events – treatment is about targets, numbers, what donors like."

Analysts agree that, despite its immense promise, the initial constituency for HIV prevention was not powerful enough to compete with those advocating care, treatment, and research (Bowtell, 2007). It is said that the "care and treatment coalition" determines priorities as these constituencies arrange conferences and thereby affect much more effectively politicians, donors, and the public debate about the distribution of limited resources. By its nature, those who used to adamantly advocate prevention were not as well represented in the higher echelons of the AIDS business, and this despite the fact that the constituency of those at risk of HIV infection is far greater than those who require ART. Bowtell (2007) is of the opinion that prevention did not feature prominently on the HIV and AIDS agenda given the fact that the political benefits of pursuing this approach are negligible. For Bowtell, "the urgent has trumped the important and generated a peculiar but real moral hazard."

Peter Piot (2008) equally cautioned that we could not continue with unabated treatment, as he indicated that for every one person treated with ART, five to six people are newly infected with the disease.

Farmer et al. (2000) suggest that prevention can be divided into primary and secondary preventions. Primary prevention is about preventing people from infection in the first place, while secondary prevention concerns preventing those infected from HIV progression (Farmer et al., 2000). Globally, the focus is mostly on secondary prevention, as can be witnessed by the rapidity and success of rolling out ART all over the world, not to mention the triumphant ART narrative in South Africa. Since 2012, primary prevention has also been officially medicalized with the Food and Drug Administration (FDA)'s approval of pre-exposure prophylaxis (PrEP) or chemoprophylaxis against HIV infection. This has been designed for use by HIV-negative individuals at high risk of contracting HIV (such as men who have sex with men (MSM), sex workers, and sero-discordant couples). The commercialized name of PrEP is Truvada, produced by the pharmaceutical company Gilead Sciences and comprises a combination of tenofovir and emtricitabine. Its initial success was established after the iPrex trial conducted in 2010 that led to the FDA's 2012 approval.[8] Not to be confused with "Treatment as Prevention"[9] (TasP), PrEP involves *non-infected people* taking treatment in order to ward off potential infection, focusing on "at-risk" or "most-at-risk" groups in particular, as a potentially dangerous cohort for future infection. Therefore, even in the domain of prevention that used to rely on social or behavioral interventions or transformations, the focus has shifted to a biomedical narrative, finally to tell a more successful tale of prevention. In the South African context, there is strong support for PrEP with published articles that act as guidance for the adoption of PrEP (Bekker et al., 2012). Access to PrEP to those most at risk of being infected was hailed by Chris Beyrer, president of the International AIDS Society in his plenary speech at the 7th South African AIDS Conference in June 2015 as "prevention equity." He, therefore, urged WHO to express stronger leadership with regard to PrEP and appealed to the HIV and AIDS community to improve uptake of this new preventive measure before the next international AIDS Conference that would have taken place in Durban in 2016. His slogan, which he exhorted the audience to applaud, was "pre-exposure: it's time to deliver!" (Beyrer, 2015).

However, PrEP has also been confronted with some uncomfortable challenges – in South Africa and in the USA. Its most vociferous opponent in the USA is Michael Weinstein, the president of the US-based AIDS Healthcare Foundation who has been prominent in the fight to ensure the protection of human rights and to destigmatize HIV and AIDS in the USA since the 1980s. He has called PrEP "a public health disaster in the making" (Barro, 2014) and another HIV activist labeled PrEP as a "boutique intervention."[10] Weinstein's so-called lonely battle against PrEP revolves around the fact that he considers this intervention to be a "party drug" and key to breaking down all previous work around safety and responsibility vested in messages of condom use. His strident denial of PrEP has earned him the unenviable label of "denialist" mostly by lobbyists from the gay community, largely to discredit him and his views within the inner circles of the HIV world. Despite the vitriol of this ongoing debate, uptake of Truvada remains low in the USA (Whitaker, 2014).

As for experiences in the global South – despite the successes of trials in the USA, in the UK, and in Thailand – the VOICE (Vaginal and Oral Interventions to Control the Epidemic) trail that was conducted in South Africa and Uganda resulted in disappointing and unexpected outcomes. In this trial, as well as the FEM PrEP trial, some of the interventions had to be stopped due to their futility and similar outcomes compared to placebo cohorts (Marazzo et al., 2015). In fact, it was ascertained that the women in these studies, given the pharmacokinetic evidence, did not take their PrEP medication (tablets or gels) as prescribed, although they reported that they did, and their pill counts indicated as much. This led to a qualitative study, VOICE C, which aimed to ascertain the reasons why study participants will go to these lengths to "misrepresent" their conduct, and by doing so, using "elaborate deceptions"[11] (McNeil, 2015a) to persuade the researchers that they were adhering to their trial medication. This obviously raises ethical questions not only about the conduct of these types of trials but also about the use of PrEP in a context such as South Africa. First, conducting such trials now requires much more frequent blood tests, and questions abound as to the incentive that payments bring into the equation of participating in this type of study. Although a negligible US$10–US$15 per visit to the clinic has been debated, it can nevertheless act as a reason for women to join the study. Then, there is also the issue of providing free healthcare services and contraception. In settings where stigma around HIV abounds, taking ART, even for prevention, was equated to being HIV infected. Women seemingly did not understand the study (Van der Straten et al., 2014). In the verbatim quotes, it so happened that some did not know that their "treatments" contained ART.

In a context of a generalized HIV epidemic, PrEP is definitely more difficult to manage, seeing that a potential PrEP candidate has to be HIV negative (and remain HIV negative while on PrEP). The most important risk factor is developing resistance, and this happens especially when someone who is unknowingly HIV positive is placed on a PrEP regime. In South Africa, activists are claiming access to PrEP unreservedly (Raphael et al., 2015), and roll-out is happening at a consistent level. The efficacy of PrEP has been proven, and in South Africa, the roll-out of PrEP started among sex workers in 2016, then was made available to MSM, and young women in universities all over the country. Young out-of-school women are the most recent targeted group as from May 2018, but with seemingly low uptake as was noted after the first six months of the intervention where a mere 6% uptake was recorded (Msomi, 2019). Despite its immense potential, literature is slowly emerging that also calls on structural impediments to take up PrEP and that continue to drive such high infection rates among certain groups (Van der

Wal & Loutfi, 2017). The social challenges associated with effective uptake and use of PrEP are increasingly seen in light of the complex social landscape in which this technology is taking place, and it is even argued that a "re-branding" of PrEP might be necessary given the low uptake, especially by young women, in the first three years of its availability. Social issues of stigmatization, gender-based violence, and widespread poverty are starting to complement the mere biomedical reading of this "game changing" prevention intervention (Eakle et al., 2018).

Resources exceptionalism

Second, and in line with Smith and Whiteside's (2010) taxonomy, HIV exceptionalism resides in its disease-specific global response. HIV exceptionalism is, therefore, also criticized from this point of view: the so-called AIDS industry, spearheaded by UNAIDS, has witnessed scathing critique from a vocal source, Roger England (2008) who is of the opinion that although HIV is a major disease in sub-Saharan Africa, it does not pose a "global catastrophe." He, therefore, deeply criticizes as mere sensationalism the language that circulates among those active in the AIDS industry who describe this epidemic as "one of the make-or-break forces of this century" and as harboring a "potential threat to the survival and well-being of people worldwide." He continues by condemning the large sums of money that he sees to have been "wasted" on inefficient programs to address HIV and AIDS. This wastage of resources England reckons was also misused by funding "national commissions" and what he terms "esoteric disciplines and projects" instead of strengthening the abilities of public health systems to control epidemics in those areas most affected. For him, a mere 10% of the $9 billion that was normally pledged to fight HIV was actually needed for this purpose. In addition, the amount of money associated with HIV aid is often more than some countries' domestic health budgets which creates all kinds of problems, such as creating "parallel financing, employment and organizational structures" which inevitably leads to disempowering local health systems when they are most in need of robustness and independence.

Other scholars whose analyses are based on a disparaging critique of the AIDS industry reiterate England's sentiments. James Chin holds forth that AIDS activists have accepted certain myths about HIV epidemiology with the intention to maintain the disease on the political agenda and to ensure a continued flow of funding and the creation of jobs (Chin, 2006). Elizabeth Pisani (2008) is also highly critical of the masses of money that flow into maintaining the HIV agenda, and opines that this outflow of money is "rubbing out common sense." In fact, the very formation of a unique UN office to deal with matters related to HIV (UNAIDS) has been severely critiqued by Roger England (2008), creating what he calls, the "biggest vertical program in history."

In fact, England touches on the enduring paradox of global healthcare provision by highlighting the critique, at the core of AIDS exceptionalism, by calling it a "vertical program." A vertical program is focused only on one disease, whereas a horizontal program seeks to strengthen the myriad of aspects that actually synergistically make up a health system. The debate around vertical and horizontal healthcare interventions and programs is a seemingly endless debate. As I will explain in Chapter 3, the entire Community Health Worker question revolves around this question: should these health workers be employed to narrowly address a bouquet of health issues (and correspond to a more vertical intervention), or should they be mustered as change agents or advocates, who react to, and inform a wide array of health but also other social issues? The history and trajectory of primary healthcare is also steeped in these debates: the vision of primary healthcare after the Alma Ata declaration reached toward a horizontal approach, but this utopian vision of "Health for All by 2000" soon floundered given the fact that the actual mandate to achieve this goal was a largely *unfunded* project (Basilico et al., 2013; Packard, 2016).

Despite good intentions and naïve assumptions, wastage of masses of money on programs focused on HIV and AIDS inevitably took place over the years. This funding often happened because those in power could prioritize their own convictions. A case in point has been that money allocated from the PEPFAR programs were, in fact, proven to have been wasted as they were focused on abstinence programs only (Piot, 2008). Helen Epstein (2007) argues that in Uganda, the widely praised decrease in HIV infection rates were linked directly to the locally conceived prevention program based on reducing multiple concurrent sexual partners, titled "Zero Grazing." Epstein is of the opinion that the PEPFAR programs with their message of abstinence caused more harm than good in this context, where a public health policy already existed and was context specific but was replaced by a more generic version that did not take into account local expertise and knowledge, nor its successes.

In the current context of widespread ART access, the cost of treating people, which is evidently rising with new infections and new targets, and proof that early treatment is most effective and should, therefore, be targeted, is soaring. MSF estimated that the lowest cost per patient per year for ART is US$100 (MSF 2013 in Whiteside & Strauss, 2014). This price obviously varies from one context to another, but Wilson and Fraser (2013 in Whiteside & Strauss, 2014) demonstrate the realities of these costs in South Africa. In 2012/2013, the national annual health budget was R27.5 billion. It was estimated that putting everyone with a CD4 count of 500 or less on ART would amount to R35.5 billion. If everyone who was HIV positive at that time were to be put on ART, the cost would have amounted to R43.5 billion (Whiteside & Strauss, 2014). For obvious reasons, resources exceptionalism is an issue that touches on the sensitive nerve of inequality in global relations. To give or not to give; to give more, or less; to create dependence or to respond to notions of social justice given the history of exploitation, colonialism, and unequal development, all fall within this intricate area of resources (and its problematic allocation). Allocating resources, more resources, is about more money from wealthy countries, trickling down to more needy settings, where the burdens of disease together with woefully inadequate healthcare supply are exponentially higher. It is said that global funding is increasingly directing their funding to resonate with national priorities. This surely would herald a welcome transformation that still needs to be proven and analyzed in order to measure the real effect it has on local health systems strengthening.

There are still significant amounts of money circulating in the humanitarian health and AIDS industries. In fact, the global health industry is "a multi-billion dollar enterprise," and the current level at which global health initiatives are operating at is unprecedented (Packard, 2016). However, despite this unparalleled scale and complexity of global health actions, Randall Packard (2016) reminds us that the "central motivations, organizing principles, and modes of operation" that today describe global health's stretch are features that are not new. Packard's enquiry in his book on the history of global health is to try and decipher the reasons why, despite the investment of billions of dollars in efforts to improve global health, some issues were not analyzed or ignored altogether, to make sense of the global (mal)distribution of ill health and bad health intervention outcomes. These neglected issues, he claims, are "basic health services, public health infrastructure, and the underlying social and economic determinants of ill health" (Packard, 2016). These issues mentioned are mostly those that characterize horizontal health programmatic interventions and approaches and again point to the extreme faith that has historically been invested rather into "magic bullet," quick-fix, vertical programs to respond to the health needs especially in those areas (the global South) where disease and disaster strike most intensely.

Rights exceptionalism

The responses to HIV and AIDS since its first identification in the 1980s were largely shaped by activism; activism that was borne out of a deep-felt necessity that HIV was different. Strong voices emerged globally to advocate for the rights of those infected as was witnessed by organizations such as the New York's Gay Men's Health Crisis that was founded as early as 1981. In the UK, the Terrence Higgins Trust was the first organization of this kind that was created in 1983, whereas France saw its activist group called AIDES come into being in 1984. In 1986, the Global Network of People Living with HIV/AIDS (GNP+), first known as the International Steering Committee of People living with HIV/AIDS, was created as a voice for PLWHAs across national borders. The well-known US activist group, Act Up (The AIDS Coalition to Unleash Power), came into existence in 1987. As for the global South, in 1983, Brazil's gay pressure group managed to advocate for the implementation of the first government AIDS program in São Paolo State. Uganda's famous TASO (The AIDS Support Organization) saw the light as early as 1987, while South Africa's Treatment Action Campaign (TAC) was formed in 1998.

The road to access treatment was difficult and unstable, to say the least. At first, activists lobbied for general access to the single-dose AZT that was administered at first to somehow halt the progression of the disease within bodies. Then happened the announcement at the 1996 International AIDS Conference in Vancouver where combination protease inhibitor treatment marked the potential end of inevitable AIDS deaths, as it could now become a manageable, chronically managed disease like many others. The costs associated with this treatment was still, however, prohibitively expensive. This "protease moment" denoted the beginning of a protracted and intense movement of fluctuating successes toward global ART access.

The "activist" turn of this disease was also evident in testing for HIV. This testing has been available since 1985 but even today is still not treated like any other testing for disease. There has always been a strong emphasis on informed consent and on pre- and post-counseling in the testing spectrum, which sets HIV apart from other diagnoses such as those of STDs (syphilis or Hepatitis B). In many instances, it has been shown that HIV testing and potential diagnosis is actively avoided, even with the availability of lifesaving treatment (De Cock et al., 2002).

Today, there is no reason why HIV could not be a chronic and manageable ailment. Despite the development in HIV treatment, AIDS advocacy remains locked in a discourse on rights and its often-unwitting consequence, internalized stigma. This has bred an entrenched HIV exceptionalism – an attitude of treatment and handling of HIV as a different and "extraordinary" case compared to tuberculosis (TB), diabetes, or hypertension, among others – to the detriment, some argue, of collective public health rights. In fact, De Cock et al. (2002) are of the opinion that "public health and human rights were portrayed as polarized and even conflicting." The message, internalized and repeated *ad infinitum* by South Africans adhering to their treatment is that HIV is like any other disease, diabetes being an oft-mentioned example. This is the message conveyed during drug readiness training, a compulsory course that all identified ART users in the public sector have to undergo before the onset of treatment. HIV being similar to other diseases could and should be the case, but getting the HIV test done is definitely not similar to being diagnosed with a disease, such as diabetes or TB.

As De Cock et al. (2002) argue, HIV exceptionalism or, to be more specific, HIV rights exceptionalism became the global norm as very little or no debate whatsoever took place in countries with exceptionally high rates of infection as to the manner in which testing should be presented and proposed to patients. This is an interesting remark, given the strong resemblances between TAC's *modus operandi* in South Africa, and the legendary Act Up that paved the way for AIDS activism, first in the USA and subsequently in other countries too. Peter Piot (2008) has referred to TAC as "a worldwide leader in activism today," following as energetically in the passionate and dedicated struggle that characterized Act Up's activities. The TAC's successes and constant reinvention are treated in Chapter 4, but of interest here are

their origins and their emphasis on human rights. By comparing the documentaries of the two organizations – *United in Anger. A History of Act Up*
(released in 2012) and the TAC's documentary *Taking HAART* (released in
2011),[12] it can be deduced that the South African activist group's fight for
biomedical intervention, its language of human rights and social justice, and
inevitably its initial adoption of "diffidence to HIV testing" (De Cock et al.,
2002) originated in the time-specific context of the USA. This era in the
USA marked a time when very little was known about the pathogenesis and
evolution of HIV, when treatment was totally unavailable, and when the
disease struck sub-populations of gay men and intravenous drug users that
inevitably provided moralists with unprecedented ammunition to discrim-
inate against these already stigmatized groups (De Cock et al., 2002). The
same context can be sketched for the early years of the South African AIDS
epidemic: unavailability of generalized treatment, widespread discrimination
and fear related to infection and the consequences of the disease, and then
the unprecedented battle against AIDS denialism, personified by the former
President Thabo Mbeki and his then Minister of Health, the late Manto
Tshabalala-Msimang.

This exceptional nature of HIV, which saw the creation in the USA of an
interesting mix of activists (gay men, medical and public health specialists,
civil liberties proponents) brought about a strong lobby group to counter
prevention methods that might have "driven the epidemic underground"
(Bayer, 1991), such as quarantine, compulsory testing and disclosure, and an
AIDS registry. Therefore, in this context, individual human rights of those
infected were framed to outmaneuver consequentialist, utilitarian public
health practices that were widely exercised and accepted. The rationalistic
and biomedical manner in which politicians, bureaucrats, and the medical
world responded to the disease also solicited an unprecedented wave of activism that took root globally in the early years of the epidemic in order to contest the discriminatory representations of the disease and the stigmatization
of already marginalized people. Act Up's members, as was the case with the
TAC, fought their respective governments for their perceived reluctance to
act in the face of a mounting epidemic.[13] An interviewee refers to the USA's
health policies of "medical apartheid," and members of Act Up are shown
storming and occupying the FDA and National Institutes of Health (NIH)
headquarters to demand access to treatment and to speed up processes around
authorization of medication. In a similar vein, the TAC's activism around
treatment was unprecedented, *with and against* the government of the new
South Africa,[14] winning a number of prominent court cases to secure the
provision of ART to expectant mothers and their babies, to inmates, and to
the public through public healthcare facilities.

This activism, originating in the USA, first led to HIV being treated as
different, as exceptional, as reinventing public health responses to an infectious disease. HIV never became a notifiable disease. It led to HIV tests always being accompanied by pre- and post-counseling. It led to the scrapping

of case detections and population screenings and required fully fledged informed consent from the potential patient to test for HIV infection. It is, therefore, argued by some that this register of exceptionality exacerbated HIV-related stigma as the disease was, from the outset, shrouded in secrecy, mystery, anonymity, and otherness. By challenging classical approaches to epidemic control, some critics foresaw a potential disaster as this disease's unique representation.

The positive contributions of AIDS activism, in the USA as in South Africa, the selfless efforts and years of hard, physical labor of meeting, marching, fighting, and persevering in the face of danger and death were instrumental in shaping AIDS responses and averting even more deaths and afflictions. However, should the question of testing have been confronted differently? Would another, more context-specific approach have made a difference to the still widespread phenomenon of stigma,[15] especially in countries in sub-Saharan Africa where HIV is different inasmuch as it is a generalized, heterosexually transmitted epidemic?

Moralistic exceptionalism

> It is all the more urgent, given the propensity of medical facts to generate highly moralistic emotions, imbued with notions of responsibility and blame, and bearing the potential to mark or single out particular social actors as loci of responsibility. A history of the present may make these facts, seemingly ineluctable, appear as *one* potential means of framing a problem within a larger field of possibilities.
>
> (Race, 2001)

Moralistic discourses around HIV and AIDS are rife and multiple. This fourth register encompasses the fact that HIV is largely spread through intimate sexual exchanges, and to a lesser extent, using recreational drugs. The uncomfortable domain of the private and intimate has to be voyeuristically exposed, analyzed and objectified, and subjected to control and prescription.[16] The rights discourses were aimed specifically to challenge the high-minded and self-righteous premonitions and recommendations that continue despite very real progress that has been made to normalize the lives of those infected with HIV. The rights discourse also attempted to break away from the overly moralistic framing of the disease.

Origins of a dreaded disease: in search of a culprit

For a long time, the starting point of the AIDS conversation was animated by the origins of AIDS. The zoonotic origins of HIV, where humans were somehow infected with an "ancestral retrovirus derived from the Simian Immunodeficiency virus present in wild chimpanzee populations in the Congo River basin" (Yusim, 2001 in Nguyen & Sama, 2008), set the tone to identify the origin of the dreaded affliction and led to speculations as to the manner in which this epidemic was spread in the first place. As demonstrated by Patton (1990a), a 1989 article in the revered *Social Science & Medicine* by authors Rushton and Bogaert, applied sociobiology, which was at the time, the most influential form of genetic logic, to convince,

> That race *per se*, as a marker of genetically determined intelligence level, degree of sexual control, and social organization ought to be considered a risk factor in the transmission of HIV. Having "established" the genetically linked lower intelligence of "negroids" and accepted as agreed that "within the constraints allowed by the total spectrum of cultural alternatives, people create norms and environments maximally compatible with their genotypes," Rushton and Bogaert argue that lowered levels of intelligence must also be considered a risk factor. Observation of contingent danger may be less, both in terms of acquiring the disease, and in transmitting it to others. There are many problems in Africa in educating people to avoid intercourse with prostitutes, or other at risk behaviors such as scarification, tattooing, ear piercing, male or female circumcision, blood-brotherhood ceremonies, etc.
>
> (Patton, 1990a)

Patton's article, *Inventing "African AIDS"* (Patton, 1990a), is an echo of the acclaimed rendition of V.Y. Mudimbe's *The Invention of Africa: Gnosis, Philosophy and the Order of Knowledge* (Mudimbe, 1988). Many other authors, like Richard and Rosalind Chirimuuta, Virginia van der Vliet, Paula Treichler, and Simon Watney, offer accounts of the manner in which HIV and AIDS fortified existing prejudices that were harbored *vis-à-vis* Africans and Africa as a continent (Chirimuuta & Chirimuuta, 1987; Treichler, 1989; Watney, 1989; Van der Vliet, 2001). African practices, culturally determined by knowledge, attitudes, behavior, and practices (KABP) studies, the manner in which AIDS and its clinical symptoms could be traced to local understandings of the body, of sexuality, of death, and interests in "exotic sexual rites" and African "sexual systems," and Africans' contact with non-human primates, all conspired to construct "African AIDS."

Only slowly and partially did this focus on culture and difference give way to more inquiry related to the political economy of HIV and AIDS (Nguyen & Sama, 2008). This new approach to looking into notions of poverty and conceding the fact that poverty leads to higher levels of vulnerability to be infected and affected by HIV at times had another outcome, "sometimes culminating into individualistic accounts or 'culture of poverty' accounts" (Geshekter, 1995 in Sama & Nguyen, 2008). It was, and still is, difficult to move beyond moralistic discourses when HIV and AIDS is at stake. In fact, Epstein and Packard (in Sama & Nguyen, 2008) cautioned early in the history of the disease that political and economic determinants will have to be taken seriously in order to truly understand the complexities around HIV.

Ignoring these structural issues, they argued, would lead to individuals being held responsible for conditions over which they had very restricted agency.

Zoning into MARPs

Specific groups of people are overly affected by HIV infection and related AIDS morbidity and mortality. These groups "most at risk" are normally already under suspicion in normative societies: MSM,[17] sex workers, intravenous drug users, but also heterosexual "black" people in light of the depictions of "African AIDS" that proliferated in popular and academic texts in the early years of the epidemic. Judgments were readily cast about people's sexual practices and preferences, and some analysts deem that this took place in lieu of the necessary frank talk that was needed to adequately address more realistic modes of transmission. In fact, Helen Epstein (2007) identified concurrent sexual partnering in hyper-epidemic countries as one of the main drivers of the epidemic. She is of the opinion that such social sensitive issues were not addressed in an adequate manner despite all the resources that were invested into addressing the epidemic.

Discourses of blame have gradually shifted to emphasize the manner in which focused care and prevention among MARPs might be able to make significant inroads in curbing new infection rates but also to somehow respond to issues of social justice, given who these specific groups comprise of. Blaming becomes morally more complex in contexts of generalized epidemics, where MARPs are, for example, young women. During his speech at the 7th South Africa AIDS Conference in Durban in 2015, the then Deputy President Cyril Ramaphosa displaced the blame when speaking about South Africa's epidemiological reality. He noted that in South Africa, one in four new infections takes place in women aged 14–24 and added that

> We must confront the reality that the astonishingly high infection rates among young South African women has much to do with the behaviour of men. It has much to do with how men of that age – and older – relate to women. It has much to do with the forms that social interaction takes and how sexual relations are conducted. It calls for greater awareness, greater respect and greater responsibility.
>
> (Ramaphosa, 2015)

Although young women comprise the biggest cohort of MARP in South Africa, men are singled out for their behavior, sexually and medically, in the context of African AIDS.

Men also register poorer outcomes in terms of treatment, as was underscored by Beyrer (2015) during his plenary speech at the 7th South African AIDS Conference. He cited more examples related to this problem: worldwide, men make up only 41% of those receiving ART. In their first year of being on ART, men are also 40% more likely to die. These gender differences in terms of treatment and treatment success seemingly persist throughout the treatment course, and Beyrer concluded that a systematic review found no interventions targeting men on the treatment cascade, thus making men on ART, a MARP.

A more unexpected MARP has been singled out to be transgender women, and it was reported that HIV most disproportionally affects this group, although no data on this sub-population exist in the African context (Beyrer, 2015). During another plenary by Zethu Matebeni (2015), she referred to lesbian and transgender women as being a group overlooked after more than 20 years of campaigns and research. Transphobia has not been widely addressed, especially in the African context, to grapple with the experiences of this newly identified MARP in sub-Saharan Africa.

Despite this seemingly positive shift in the discourse of MARPs, sex workers and MSM are still criminalized in many settings around the globe. The criminalization of HIV is still rife and, therefore, inevitably drives the epidemic underground, to use the ubiquitous phrase that served as justification to approach HIV and AIDS differently in the first place and to largely foil conventional public health procedures. The moralistic tendencies that accompany the (inevitable) representations of MARPs are, therefore, problematic as new infections continue unabated despite processes of normalization.

The securitization and criminalization of HIV

In 2000, a speech by the then US Vice President, Al Gore at the UN Security Council, highlighted this disruptive potential of HIV if left unchecked,

> It [HIV] threatens not just individual citizens, but the very institutions that define and defend the character of a society … It strikes at the military, and subverts the forces of order and peacekeeping.
>
> (Gore, 2000)

The UN Security Council decided to pass Resolution 1308, which states, "The illness poses a risk to stability and security." In addition, the US National Intelligence Council produced "The Global Infectious Disease Threat and Its Implications for the United States" (US National Intelligence Council, 2000). In South Africa, the Institute for Security Studies issued a report that alerted to the potential threatening effects of HIV and that it "could hinder the processes of democratization by undermining social development and intensifying the struggle for resources" (Pharaoh & Schonteich, 2003).

"AIDS orphans" were also a topic of discussion in this report to the extent that they could contribute to social disruption,

> Bluntly put, those who are orphaned may be indifferent to prevailing norms and values, may look for salvation to millenarian and fundamentalist beliefs of one kind or another, and may ultimately do this with assistance from a Kalashnikov or a bomb.
>
> (Barnett & Whiteside, 2002)

This new focus on security related to AIDS and its potential impacts on orphans and the threat of terror began to inhabit the imagination of many despite the lack of evidence to prove these unsubstantiated fears (Barnett & Prins, 2006). HIV, untreated, and largely limited to the developing, third world or the global South, was still powerfully perceived as a virus that could have far-reaching consequences for the rich and powerful, even though these developed, first world countries' risk of infection and disease proliferation had significantly declined (Smith & Whiteside, 2010).

In some instances, HIV infection is still framed in an accusatory manner and as an individual's sole responsibility. This register can be expanded to include issues of HIV and criminalization from a range of perspectives, including penalties related to known infection and undisclosed, unprotected, sexual relations and criminalization of MSM, sex workers, and intravenous drug users. Knight (2006) indicates offending examples of international reactions to PLWHAs. The President of the German Federal Court of Justice stated that it might become mandatory to tattoo or to quarantine these individuals, but this suggestion was fortunately never endorsed. Also in Germany, those applying for extended residency permits in Bavaria needed to undergo an HIV test. In China and in India, HIV testing used to be compulsory for all foreign visitors entering these countries for over one year and all returning citizens. The US Senate also voted unanimously to decree HIV tests for those applying for legal immigration. Some countries in South and South-East Asia followed these examples and introduced similar actions (Knight, 2006). In an article appearing in 2009 (Zaheer et al., 2009 in Whiteside, 2009), it was indicated that 85 UN member countries criminalize sex between adults of the same gender and that in ten of these countries, the state has the power to impose the death penalty in instances where this law is breached. In many countries, injecting drug use and sex work are criminalized. Given these punitive laws, these groups remain generally inaccessible to conventional public health services (Zaheer et al. 2009 in Whiteside, 2009). According to more recent statistics, some 61 countries still have legislation entrenched that permits the criminalization of HIV non-disclosure, exposure, or transmission. UNAIDS also indicated that in 76 countries, same-sex sexual activities are still being criminalized, and that in seven countries, these deeds are punishable by death (UNAIDS, 2015b).

Criminalization and moralizing lead to some seriously flawed public health decisions, where in a country like Ghana, with a 78% HIV prevalence among sex workers and sex workers accounting for 76% of transmission sources, 99.2% of funding is targeted at the general population and, therefore, not at sex workers (Whiteside, 2009). Criminalization is not unique to Africa, though. When HIV first appeared to be a problem in the early 1980s in the USA, and when infections started mounting in other parts of the world, notably in the developing world, the disease was depicted as posing a real threat to security in the developed world, and a discourse of securitization was developed in order to justify actions and interventions to fight this new scourge (Penfold, 2015).

The domain of the moralistic is riddled with obstacles. It might be one reason among many others that our focus on prevention is not that well articulated. This might be because prevention – as has been shown by Helen Epstein's (2007) account of Uganda's "zero grazing" policy – is, at times, closely linked to behavioral approaches, which have a very close resemblance to forms of moralizing. To dictate to people how they should lead their lives, especially their sexual lives, is always problematic. Have we, as social and cultural scientists, broached the topics of sexuality and morality adequately, or has our "treading-on-eggs" approach around sexuality and Africa – because of the many impasses of the past – been, ironically, also exoticized? Recently, more accounts of a growing responsibilization of sexual practices, especially issues pertaining to disclosure to sexual partners, are seeing the day (Young, 2015). Has the important focus on structural issues obscured the other, equally important part of the equation, i.e. taking responsibility for one's sexual actions?

African and South African exceptionalism

> While this case of high-level political interference in the scientific arena may appear extreme and exceptional, it nonetheless draws attention to more general questions relating to science, politics and citizenship in the 21st century.
>
> (Robins, 2004)

The year 2001 saw an exceptional gathering of 45 heads of state of the then Organization of African Unity (currently known as the African Union) to break the silence surrounding HIV and AIDS. This exceptional meeting led to the 2001 Abuja Declaration on HIV and AIDS, where African leaders pledged their commitment to fighting the scourge by dedicating agreed percentages of their gross domestic product toward AIDS funding.

Despite this unequivocal declaration, controversies, debates, and accusations around HIV and Africa were and still are plentiful. First, linking HIV's origins to Africa seemed to occupy an important causative explanation, linking African sexuality, more so, promiscuity, to the proliferation of the disease in Africa and elsewhere. Many authoritative analyses have plotted this discourse from various angles, mostly by quoting former President Mbeki's acerbic statement during the 2001 Z.K. Matthews memorial speech delivered at the Fort Hare University[18]:

> Thus does it happen that others who consider themselves to be our leaders take to the streets carrying their placards to demand that because we [black people] are germ carriers, and human beings of a lower order that cannot subject its [sic] reason to passion we must perforce adopt strange opinions, to save a depraved and diseased people from perishing from self-inflicted disease... convinced that we are but natural-born

promiscuous carriers of germs ... they proclaim that our continent is doomed to an inevitable mortal end because of our devotion to the sin of lust.

(Mbeki, 2001)

Directly after the emergence of AIDS, the overwhelming concern of social scientists was to venture into explaining the skyrocketing HIV prevalence in terms of "African specificities" (Sama & Nguyen, 2008) and, as I have indicated earlier, by "othering" African sexual practices. This type of enquiry has largely subsided in the new period of medicalization, and we have come a long way since the dark days of Mbeki-era "denialism," despite some deeply discomforting accuracies it pointed out. The incidence of what is known as South African "denialism" or the "Mbeki era" resonated globally as an inconceivable response to a rampant HIV and AIDS epidemic within the country. This episode in South Africa's history dramatized and exceptionalized the epidemic even more. The then Minister of Health, Dr. Aaron Motsoaledi, refers to this period as the "lost decade" within the history of HIV.[19] In light of the systematic refusal of government to provide HIV treatment in the public sector, we witnessed the emergence of the most pronounced activist activity post-apartheid with the creation of TAC in 1998 to fight for universal access to ART. Globally funded programs and humanitarian aid interventions in developing countries, and a more HIV-orthodox government (in South Africa, after the end of Thabo Mbeki's presidency) led to the slow introduction of HAART into these HIV-burdened areas within the developing world.

The increased availability of ART in the public healthcare sector led to the increase of exceptional outcomes as patients in South Africa performed exceptionally well on treatment and achieved a remarkable adherence rate. Numerous accounts of "near death" experiences that were thwarted by this "magical" treatment are told, and miraculous, Lazarus–tales started populating popular media and academic discourses simultaneously. The fight for HAART started for those who still did not have access to this lifeline. The stark inequalities that subsequently characterized the disease were positioned as the new reality of the HIV and AIDS epidemic. Patents, prices, and politicians were at the forefront of keeping lifesaving treatment from those in dire need thereof.

I indicated that South Africa, for a variety of reasons, manifests as an exceptional example of a unique disease emergence, as well as of distinctive responses to HIV and AIDS. The most flagrant example was its HIV emergence on the heels of South Africa's historical trajectory of a unique dispensation of racially based colonial rule despite widespread changes on the African continent as from the 1960s (Seidman, 1999). As Seidman explains, the country used to be exemplary for its global pariah status, but since 1994 became distinguished in terms of its exemplarity: the rather peaceful end to years of apartheid and associated racial oppression and the "new" South Africa became a crucible for potential positive transformations. Then AIDS happened. For yet another reason, South Africa became a familiar name globally, and this time because of its unprecedented HIV and AIDS epidemic. Didier Fassin (2002) broaches this South African exceptionalism by referring to both the "uniqueness" and "exemplarity" of South African AIDS. By *uniqueness*, he specifically refers to the historical context in which HIV took root: the specific political context, past and present, first characterized by racial segregation and systemized discrimination, which still resonate in the unequal and discriminatory manner in which HIV and AIDS disproportionately affects the very population groups that also bore the brunt of apartheid. In his emphasis on *exemplarity*, on the other, he explains the manner in which structural realities, in South Africa as elsewhere, are closely related to the "dynamic of diseases" (Fassin, 2002). Under the rubric of "uniqueness," Fassin equally mentions the political interference in the handling of AIDS, embodied in the Mbeki-era denialism and the former president's search for "African solutions to African problems" being the overarching theme of a host of bizarre events that grabbed the attention of academics, scientists, ordinary people and charlatans[20] worldwide. However, this phenomenon of denialism sadly came at a huge cost in terms of human lives.[21] The statistics were staggering: during the height of AIDS denialism in 2002/2003, when the then Minister of Health, Manto Tshabalala-Msimang considered that AIDS did not deserve special attention, more than 25% of the adult population and more than 11% of the total population were HIV positive. In 2002 alone, more than 360,000 people died of AIDS-related conditions, it was estimated that 660,000 children were orphaned during this period of time, and every day saw 1,500 more people being newly infected (Van Niekerk, 2014). This exceptionality was compounded by another sobering fact: South Africa soon became the country in the world with the highest number of HIV-positive individuals.

Since 2004, and a change in political leadership, under the tutelage of Dr. Motsoaledi, South Africa boasts the world's largest ART program. In fact, at the closing plenary of the 7th South African AIDS Conference, in light of critique related to drug stock-outs (of which ARTs)[22] and deficient healthcare in public facilities, Dr Motsoaledi, after a verbose explanation that stock-outs could, in effect, not be occurring, declared that the ART program will fail "over my dead body." He mentioned several solutions, of which many include the use of new technology, to track drug stock-outs in clinics, and explained that each clinic in KwaZulu Natal – one of South Africa's nine provinces – has a designated cellphone with an app that is used to monitor drug stock-outs. An eloquent and detailed description of his handling of the drug stock-outs ensued, ending on the high note that 90% of all South Africans on ART are on a fixed-dose combination (FDC) and that all depots had a 10% buffer stock of these pills. He referred to the unavoidable logistical errors that can occur at local levels and said that it is to be expected that the country, which hosts 30% of the world's ART program, would experience some anomalies. Pleading with facilities not to allow patients to leave without medication, he said, "You can go to the press, but help the patients first."

South Africa's exceptional status related to HIV and AIDS has undergone a massive transformation over the years, from the "lost" to the so-called "lax" years. We are now in a register of exceptionality that is commendable and orthodox compared to the years of denialism and heterodoxy that marked the early 2000s. However, the government should perhaps pay heed to the accusations from activists as to a perceived slackening in their attitude toward health-related issues. Although it might be ridiculous to call Dr Motsoaledi a "denialist," especially in light of the evocative nature of this appellation, the future is difficult to foretell, and current decisions and choices might become tomorrow's scapegoat.

Notes

1　Chris Hani was an anti-apartheid freedom fighter who was also the leader of the South African Communist Party. He was assassinated in 1993.
2　HIV was discovered as the likely cause of AIDS first by Luc Montagnier of the Pasteur Institute in France and subsequently by Robert Gallo of the National Institutes of Health (USA) in 1984. However, medical practitioners in other countries realized that they had been treating this disease since the 1970s and earlier. The link between the so-called slim disease present in parts of Africa and the first cases of AIDS or GRID (gay-related immunodeficiency syndrome) was made in the early 1980s. However, the early years of the disease were characterized by widespread denial that this infection could become a heterosexual problem or for that matter, a generalized, global public health concern.
3　Two well-known HIV experts, Tony Barnett and Alan Whiteside, expanded on the term "long-wave event" to explain the appearance of AIDS and its complex implications (Barnett & Whiteside, 2002). The term was originally coined by Barnett and Blaikie (1990), and has since the advent of ART been under renewed scrutiny to make sense of the changing face of HIV as a chronic condition.
4　Cindy Patton, in her much-cited work published in 1990 on the invention of African AIDS, cautions that: "Linking disease and poverty in a simple fashion leaves the way open to the unconscious reflex of westerners to situate *poverty* as well as disease in the context of racial/ethnic difference rather than in larger world-wide patterns of colonialism, capitalist statism, and a global economy increasingly in the control of supranational corporations" (Patton, 1990a). Nevertheless, in his controversial outbursts during the years of AIDS denialism, Mbeki surely also incorporated this latter part explaining the spread of HIV in South Africa.
5　"Universal access" to ART is broadly defined as aiming for high levels of access that is affordable (80% or more of the eligible population). It, therefore, does not entail 100% coverage (World Health Organization, 2015b).
6　These ambitious targets, according to the South African Ministry of Health, are also valid and have been adopted for the equally vexing problem of tuberculosis (TB). The HIV epidemic and the TB scourge thrive in each other's company, and have been dubbed "the terrible twins." As the less appealing twin in the couple, TB care and policy implementation have been severely neglected in South Africa, which now witnesses an alarming increase in MDR TB (multiple drug resistant TB) and even XDR TB (extensively drug resistant TB).
7　The UNAIDS postcard that was distributed at the 7th South African HIV/AIDS Conference frames these targets as "an ambitious treatment target to help end the AIDS epidemic," and this is also the title of UNAIDS' report.

8 PROUD and IPERGAY were two trials that were both terminated early given the undisputed efficacy of PrEP, even used with different dosages in the two trials.

9 The Trial HPTN052's report released in 2015 indicated the sustained benefit of early HIV treatment to reduce further HIV infections.

10 This utterance was apparently made during the CROIC conference in Boston in 2011 (INCIDENCE, 2014).

11 Cindy Patton (1990a) refers to this not as deception, but rather as "dual discourse competence," used *vis-à-vis* Western science and professed rationality to "defend, deflect, appease."

12 TAC explicitly adopted the activist model developed by Act Up with its emphasis on "treatment literacy" among people who are directly implicated by the disease. In 1999, Act Up came to South Africa to provide training to the first cohort of treatment literacy activists (Heywood, 2009).

13 The documentaries are similar in as much as staggering statistics are graphically and unequivocally displayed: In *United in Anger*, the message of AIDS deaths is the leitmotiv of the documentary with a digital screening that during a given amount of seconds, someone had died of HIV because of the issue of non-access to treatment. In the TAC's version, the recurrent digitally displayed message contrasted the number of South Africans infected in a given year with the number of people who have died, and lastly indicating the slow initial progress of the number of people accessing treatment in the same year. The curves show a telling tale of skyrocketing infections and deaths and a flat line indicating access to ART from 2003 to 2009 within South Africa.

14 In 2000, the South African government, thanks to the support of TAC as *amicus curiae*, won the landmark case against the 49 pharmaceutical companies (represented by the Pharmaceutical Manufacturers Association) who opposed the amendments of the Medicines Act (amendments related to the manufacture and import of generic medicines in order to provide more affordable drugs to South Africans). This was the one and only form of litigation that united the government and TAC. Thereafter, a string of litigations followed in which TAC took on the South African authorities. The most famous cases are the 2001/2002 victory of TAC requiring the government to start with a prevention-of-mother-to-child program and the 2004 ground-breaking triumph to force government to implement a national ARV program.

15 The Stigma Index Study, a study conducted among 10,000 PLWHA in South Africa in 2014, the findings of which were launched in 2015, indicates that internalized stigma is the most prevalent form of stigma among PLWHA (Human Sciences Research Council, 2015).

16 Cindy Patton (1990a) traces some of these uncomfortable intimate hypotheses, especially related to Africa, and she argues that they were constructed by racist and homophobic Western medicine to prove "otherness" – hypotheses that were often to be proven wrong.

17 Chris Beyrer indicated that there are worrying increases in HIV infection among MSM in China, Thailand, and Kenya, and among younger men in the USA, despite better lower infection rates in the USA among intravenous drug users and heterosexual people (Beyrer, 2015).

18 This quote has been used prolifically due to its immense ironic significance. Some authors, who have used this extract in their analyses of a variety of issues, are Claire Decoteau in *Ancestors and Antiretrovirals. The Bio-Politics of HIV/AIDS in post-apartheid South Africa* (Decoteau, 2013); Sylvia Tamale as the editor of *African Sexualities. A Reader* (Tamale, 2011); Rosemary Jolly's *Cultured Violence: Narrative, Social Suffering and Engendering Human Rights* (Jolly, 2010); Didier Fassin in *When Bodies Remember. Experiences and Politics of AIDS in South Africa* (Fassin,

2007); Mandisa Mbali in an article on *AIDS Discourses and the South African State* (Mbali, 2004); and in Udo Schüklenk's (2004) article titled *Professional Responsibilities of Biomedical Scientists in Public Discourse*. This list is by no means exhaustive.

19 In a play of words in the spirit of activism, some activists at the 7th South African National AIDS Conference in June 2015 refer to the current HIV climate, under the auspices of Dr Motsoaledi as the "lax decade" given its political inability to deal with some health-related problems, such as the crisis in the Free State health sector (to be discussed in Chapter 4) and treatment stock-outs in the country as a whole. The former Minister of Health is considered to not hold enough political influence to push for important health reforms in the country.

20 For an excellent account that chronicles the appearance of quackery after the emergence of HIV and AIDS, see Nathan Geffen's (2010) monograph titled *Debunking Delusions. The Inside Story of the Treatment Action Campaign*.

21 "History may judge us, the present South Africans, to have collaborated in the greatest genocide of our time by the types of choices – political or scientific – we make in relation to this HIV and AIDS epidemic." M.W. Makgoba who was the Medical Research Council President, uttered these words in 2001.

22 TAC, together with *Médecins Sans Frontières*, Section 27, Rural Doctors Association of Southern Africa, Southern Africa HIV Clinician's Society, and Rural Health Advocacy Group have already compiled two reports that deal with the exact figures and incidences of drug stock-outs within the country.

2 Dollars, donors, and drugs

South Africa in the era of global health

The invention of global health and its relation to HIV and AIDS

Given its relative youth, global health is still characterized as a field of study in the making, "more a bunch of problems than a discipline" (Kleinman, 2010). Global health's reach is impressive and its complexity even more remarkable as it conjoins efforts to improve the health of peoples all over the world with corporatism, cooperation, and the deployment of incredible resources in going about its business. Randall Packard (2016) is of the opinion that global healthcare in its current configuration is in a state of crisis and that "at its core, this history [of global health] remains predominantly about flows of goods, services, and strategies along well-trod, north-south pathways" (Packard, 2016). It was recently emphasized that even the seemingly simple process of "identifying and ranking health challenges – what historians of science call *problem choice* – demonstrates that global health priorities in the present have been patterned by social forces with roots in the colonial past" (Green et al., 2013). The ethics of global health is, therefore, increasingly under the microscope of critical social scientists in order to grasp the workings of such an ambitious, ambivalent, and multifarious undertaking as it can increasingly be read under the script of the much-scrutinized and criticized index of unfettered capitalism's neoliberal agenda.

In its charitable and altruistic resemblance to a form of humanitarianism, it makes it problematic to critique global health (Fassin, 2012a). Global health, like humanitarianism, is about alleviating suffering and saving lives, and therefore, however imperfect it might be, this form of aid is often considered better than inaction. However, the inherent contradictions or the duality of the "regimes" of global health (Lakoff, 2010) indicate that global health, with all its good and compassionate intentions, is still firmly rooted in pervasive inequalities and thrive on entrenched power imbalances. Global health, like many other humanitarian actions, is primarily about the wielding and maneuvering of political resources (Fassin, 2012b; Crane, 2013). As mentioned earlier on in the introduction, this "philanthropic industry" or "philantro-capitalism" and concomitant "disaster capitalism" are subject to increased scrutiny and critique of late. Critics of this aid approach are of the opinion that the ultimate aim of extending help and "cashing in" on disaster is about securing and strengthening the global neoliberal status quo and leaving unaddressed those structural features that are at the heart of inequalities. In Loewenstein's (2016) analysis of *Disaster Capital. Making a Killing Out of Catastrophe*, it is stated that the vulnerable in the 21st century have become a much coveted commodity in a context where the uncomfortable mix of multinational corporations, philanthropic activities, and the ill-fate of people display increasing currency to solidify yet another Janus-faced "industry," with roots firmly entrenched in existing privilege. Despite its new name, "global health" is a "mix of old and new" as it moves "back to the future" (Packard, 2016), repeating errors already committed in the past and largely disregard lessons learnt from previous failed interventions as meticulously unpacked in the work of Randall Packard (2016) that provides a history of global health. HIV and AIDS is a quintessential global health issue. This is because, first, AIDS is global in nature; it is a disease, with a spread into every country in the world. Second, its international distribution is the inevitable result of the connectivity brought about by globalization (Mbali, 2013). This chapter will deal with explaining the rise and consolidation of global health, especially with the manner in which HIV provides the formative lens through which global health has inevitably taken shape. In fact, this HIV lens and its determining role in constructing global health again points toward the exceptional status that HIV enjoyed over many years. It equally begs the question as to the future of HIV as well as global health with processes of normalization increasingly characterizing this terrain.

A quest for identity: defining global health

It is perhaps unsurprising that the term "global health" has largely been defined and developed by academics of the global North, especially North America (Crane, 2013). Johanna Crane contrasts two events, one supposedly providing evidence to the other, to agree on a "common definition of global health." She compares the actual inaugural meeting – held in 2008 of the Consortium of Universities of Global Health (CUGH) where this definition was to be discussed – with the subsequent article that ensued as a result of the conference: a piece of writing widely cited, that was published in the authoritative journal, *The Lancet*, to make public this "agreed" definition (Koplan et al., 2009). The main thrust of differentiating global health with former fields of international health,[1] tropical medicine, and colonial medicine revolved around the former's novel, "participatory' approach." This participation is not only determined in terms of the global South participating in research projects of the global North, but participation entails "the pooling of expertise and knowledge" and "a two-way flow between developed and developing countries" (Koplan et al., 2009). There is thus a sense of equality between partners from both the providers of funds and the recipients thereof. However, Crane (2013) attests to the poor representation of so-called partners emanating from the global South at this important and determining CUGH's meeting in 2008, and this to the dismay of many of the attendees. Only 4 scientists of the 50 at the CUGH's meeting were from the global South, whereas the others were all from North American institutions.[2] In fact, this terminology is used most frequently in North American settings, as can be witnessed by the salience of global health programs within North American universities. Koplan et al. (2009) state that

> Although frequently referenced, global health is rarely defined. When it is, the definition varies greatly and is often little more than a rephrasing of a common definition of public health or a politically correct updating of international health.

Lakoff (2010) conceptualizes an uncomfortable coexistence of two "regimes of global health" that are at the root of global health initiatives. First, the regime that focuses on international health security or securitization. This first register is prioritized given the porousness of global borders and the increased ease with which diseases travel from one corner of the earth to another. Adherents of this regime are, therefore, mainly concerned with the containment of the potential spread of disease. The second regime is that of compassion, humanitarianism, and the aspiration to remedy prevalent and gaping global health inequalities. This latter regime has another side, according to Crane (2013), where the compassionate impulse is paired with a "scientific mission" in as much as "international research and medical education are valorized as humanitarian endeavors ('saving lives')." The humanitarian/scientific register gives rise to the "juggernaut of activity" that we witness when it comes to the flow of money but also of bodies (those of researchers and students) from North America to Africa (not as much the other way around) in the name of humanitarian aid and of doing science. This phenomenon is referred to as "academic global health" (Crane, 2013). In fact, researchers from the global South publicly voiced their concerns about this state of affairs by stating that global health, if practiced in its current form, "risked becoming merely a means by which universities could 'brand' themselves in a competitive educational market" (MacFarlane et al., 2008, in Crane, 2013). This state of affairs could be interpreted to constitute a new form of colonization and frames global health as "an inherently postcolonial endeavor" (Crane, 2013). Crane (2013) calls this "uncomfortable mix of preventable suffering and scientific productivity," "global health science," and is of the opinion that this "global health science" ironically embodies and even gains from these inequalities that it professes to restore. Global health, in its current manifestation, is still a contested practice in terms of its ethical, political, and technical zones and its "contours are still under construction" (Lakoff, 2010).

Crane is by no means alone in voicing critique to the emergence of this new global health, seemingly different from its predecessors it supposedly improves on. Vinh-Kim Nguyen (2010) in his conceptualization of "therapeutic citizenship" also identifies the AIDS industry as increasingly entangled with development aid because of the threats that HIV and AIDS poses to economic and political futures of the globe. The global market is often structured in such a manner that the donor nations and private industries are largely in control of these initiatives. This inevitably leads to the widespread assumption that aid donors and transnational corporations have greater financial authority than most African states that are the hosts and beneficiaries of these humanitarian and scientific interventions (Poku, 2002, in Sama & Nguyen, 2008). Forms of surveillance, but also of control, thus shift from these recipient states to other entities: global, biomedical, and increasingly technical entities. These new global role players have the potential to even reconfigure the meaning of "citizenship" in as much as this concept gets increasingly expressed in terms of the biological and the medical (King, 2002; Biehl, 2004; Nguyen, 2004; Redfield, 2012).

The shift to global health from international health also witnessed a growing preference for vertical, disease-specific interventions, partially to sidestep receiving-end states with its attendant bureaucracy and the potential siphoning off of donor money by acts of corruption. In terms of HIV and AIDS, the shift to so-called verticality and the unprecedented resources provided by the wealthier parts of the world were largely welcomed by beleaguered states and their citizenry in the developing world of the global South who had no choice but to witness the slow wasting of bodies and large numbers of deaths due to AIDS. Foreign-funded interventions and research translated into new forms of healthcare provisioning (like the widespread availability of antiretroviral therapy [ART]), and allowed levels of care wholly unavailable in countries that faced high HIV infection rates.

In his analysis of discourses related to HIV and AIDS funding during the past decade, Ingram (2013) traces the declining tendency of aid. He emphasizes that a shift in focus happened from "a rationality of salvation (premised upon exception from the neoliberal norm of scarcity)" to a current discourse of "administration (premised upon the subsumption of HIV/AIDS back within a discourse of scarcity)." HIV and AIDS thus loses its "exceptional" status in this framing of continued funding requirements. Funding and aid programs become increasingly bureaucratized as there are increasing needs for "greater visibility, calculability, and attributability of all aspects of the response" and an intensification of a "discourse of scarcity (often rendered as 'sustainability')" (Ingram, 2013). Thus, it is evident that spending and funding priorities from donors all over the world are changing. HIV and AIDS funding is redirected, as witnessed in 2009 when the UK Department for International Development (DfID) redistributed some of its HIV funds to maternal and child mortality programs, as well as to health systems strengthening (PlusNews, 2009). Likewise, the Netherlands cut their spending on HIV in 2009 by US$70 million (MSF, 2009). In order to reach the end of AIDS as a public health threat by 2030, the world will have to increase HIV funding by US$1.5 billion each year between 2016 and 2020. High-income countries have decreased their HIV funding over the last couple of years, with funding dropping 7% between 2015 and 2016. Low- and middle-income countries are increasingly funding their own HIV programs. However, funding gaps put the future of HIV funding (in order to reach the 2030 goal) in a rather uncertain position (Avert, 2019). The seeming hypocrisy in the initial definition of global health as well as increased ambiguities as to the future of global health funding earmarked specifically for a wide variety of HIV endeavors are both indicative of problematic aspects of this domain of healthcare decision making. Global health and its manifestation within HIV and AIDS realities are, however, influenced to a tremendous extent by the interests and accompanying actions of people who are infected and affected by HIV (Packard, 2016).

The global response to a new scourge

> UNAIDS has made AIDS cool ... The fact that so many celebrities have been engaged with AIDS and [that] AIDS has been adopted by the culture industry has, I think, helped tremendously to de-stigmatize AIDS.
>
> (Jon Lidén, Director of Communications with
> the Global Fund, in Knight, 2006)

Fassin (2012) indicates that humanitarian politics has, on the one hand, a "long-term temporality," which relates in the main to the emergence in the 18th century onward of moral sentiments in philosophical writings and subsequently in common sense thinking and acting. On the other hand, humanitarian politics also has a "short-term temporality" which indicates concrete actions and the creation of organizations to translate these moral sentiments into tangible effects. Toward the end of the 20th century, the creation of these bodies were put in place to provide assistance in times of humanitarian need, an "industry" that has grown significantly to deal with disaster where and when it strikes in the world. This industry was configured because of the increasing spread of epidemic diseases as from the early 1990s. Another reason for the increase in action was because of the belief harbored by international donor agencies and governments that some diseases, like HIV, were intricately linked to considerable developmental downturns in resource-poor areas[3] (Packard, 2016).

The emergence of the World Health Organization (WHO) in 1948 is an example of this "short-term temporality." This organization was created by member states of the UN in response to a major cholera outbreak in Egypt that claimed roughly 20,000 lives. This organization has been responsible for important projects with impacts on a global scale. Some of the best known of these endeavors include the creation of the Model List of Essential Medicines, the Alma Ata Declaration on Primary Health Care of 1978, the 2000 Millennium Development Goals, and the more recent 2015 Sustainable Development Goals. Globally, the initial response to HIV and AIDS was apathetic, even from an organization such as the United Nations (Packard, 2016). Two WHO meetings were held in 1983 to assess the HIV and AIDS situation. The first meeting's main concern was the state of the European situation, whereas the second meeting focused on taking stock of HIV and AIDS as a global phenomenon. In the same year, an internal WHO memo indicated that there was no need for the organization to be involved in AIDS as the condition "is being well taken care of by some of the richest countries in the world where there is the manpower [sic] and the know-how and where most of the patients are to be found" (Knight, 2006). This initial delayed response to AIDS, linked largely to global denial, was admitted by the then Director-General, Halfdan Mahler,

> I know that many people at first refused to believe that a crisis was upon us. I know because I was one of them.
>
> (Mahler in Knight, 2006)

Despite this denial, the first International Conference on AIDS took place in Atlanta, Georgia, in 1985 where the focus was especially on the disease in the industrialized West. Very few African delegates were present at this conference, and "African AIDS" hardly received attention. When it did, it was mostly vested in distorted renditions and uninformed statements by renowned scientists (who grossly overestimated AIDS in Africa) and who assigned racist assumptions about African sexuality with regard to the transmission of HIV from primates to humans. Denial, accusation, and restrain thus first characterized the initial responses to AIDS in Africa. Rather slowly, as HIV infections and AIDS deaths continued at an alarming pace, more dedicated support and structures started emerging.

The attempts to create and legitimize a dedicated organization to oversee the HIV and AIDS epidemic were mired in tension and overt rivalry. The painful birth of UNAIDS in 1994/1995, and its official launch on World AIDS Day in 1995, was preceded by ideological rifts and territorial battles, especially by different co-sponsoring agencies who each at their turn claimed the AIDS agenda, notably WHO under the leadership of its then Director-General, Hiroshi Nakajimi. In fact, one of the defining ideological differences was the manner in which HIV and AIDS was to be managed. Narrowly, as a communicable disease, overseen largely by public health and epidemiology and, therefore, under the auspices of WHO. Alternatively, as envisioned by Jonathan Mann, the first Director of the first program dedicated to AIDS, the "Control Program on AIDS," set up in 1986, who viewed AIDS as a societal issue, to be coordinated and managed by various stakeholders within and outside of the UN (Knight, 2006). In between these bureaucratic infightings and competing agendas of co-sponsoring agencies, HIV infection and concomitant AIDS-related deaths continued unabatedly. After the much-disputed creation thereof, UNAIDS, under the leadership of its first Director, Peter Piot, and his team, worked tirelessly to overcome the numerous political barriers and impasses that the creation of UNAIDS gave rise to, given its unique formation as a UN agency with a range of co-sponsoring agencies, a team that comprised the secretariat, and external funders. Despite ongoing lack of coordinated support and vision among this ungainly collection of UNAIDS members, it nonetheless continued working toward a coherent response. The creation of "Theme Groups" was one of these initiatives where a range of stakeholders, including civil society members, were invited to design country-specific responses to the AIDS epidemic. UNAIDS also compiled a collection of "Best Practices" – translated into different languages – to be distributed and used in those countries hardest hit by the epidemic. Despite its contemporary critique of implementing a narrow, vertical response to but one disease, UNAIDS, from its inception, aimed at strengthening institutional capacity by introducing the "Horizontal Technical Collaboration Group" initiative to include the voices of "receiving-end" countries on issues ranging from epidemiology, care, counseling, and also national strategic planning (Packard, 2016).

At first, UNAIDS struggled to obtain the necessary legitimacy it needed as an agency to wield authority in relation to the grave state of affairs related to HIV and AIDS in the world. The conveners of the watershed 1996 International AIDS Conference in Vancouver allowed Peter Piot – only after a lot of persuasion – to address the delegates. This paved the way for UNAIDS to stake their claim as a body to be reckoned with in the HIV and AIDS community as it provided the conference with a first set of "harmonized epidemiological statistics" to reveal the extent of the disease globally (Knight, 2006). At this conference, Peter Piot was also the first UN official to publicly broach the subject of treatment access in parts of the world other than the global North. He called for access to ART to transpire as a matter of policy and called on the mobilization of such a movement. Despite the brave invitation, ART access in middle- and low-income countries would not happen for several years to come. It would emerge only after major negotiations and compromises between senior UN officials, political heavyweights, and profit-driven pharmaceutical companies, increasingly prompted by impressive and sustained activism for ART access in the global North as well as the global South.

The widespread attempts to move HIV and AIDS onto the global center stage were aided by the personal interest that the former UN Secretary-General, Kofi Annan, took in making AIDS visible by relating its devastation and impact. In June 1999, in a speech termed "The Global Challenges of AIDS," he traced the global impact of AIDS and firmly stated that AIDS is "taking away Africa's future." As Secretary-General of the UN, this was to be his first speech of many on the burning topic of HIV and AIDS (Knight, 2006; Packard, 2016). The HIV and AIDS agenda in Africa was also fortified with the signing of a Memorandum of Understanding between UNAIDS and the Organization of African Unity that stipulated collaboration and partnership in the fight against HIV and AIDS in Africa.

In these groundbreaking years of defining and framing HIV and AIDS, it sore to prominence. Security Council sessions were dedicated to discussing the multiple and far-reaching consequences of HIV, bringing HIV and AIDS to the forefront of the global political agenda. The gravity of HIV and AIDS was emphasized when a Special Session on AIDS by the UN was called: in practice, this meant that the entire UN would focus on one sole issue during a meeting, also called a UN General Assembly Special Session (UNGASS). This meeting happened in 2001 and thus put HIV and AIDS on the list of issues deemed "of the greatest global significance" (Knight, 2006). This was to be the first time a health-related issue was provided such an opportunity. In 2004 at the Copenhagen Consensus, a team of eight outstanding economists concluded that controlling HIV and AIDS should be the very first economic priority in terms of a cost-benefit analysis, not only in health but also in nutrition.

With its confidence bolstered, its legitimacy entrenched, and global acknowledgment of the impending HIV and AIDS crisis, UNAIDS started calling on more resources to meet the disease head-on. At another watershed International AIDS Conference, this time taking place in Durban, South Africa, in 2000, the first of these to happen on African soil, Piot made an historic plea to world leaders to start envision aid support in terms of billions of dollars instead of millions. He pleaded for the availability of US$3 billion a year that would have been needed to take basic measures on the continent of Africa, and another US$10 billion to provide standard ART in Africa, as was used elsewhere in the world. In addition, he called on the industrialized world to cancel the debt of African countries, with the explicit aim of using that money toward HIV and AIDS spending (Packard, 2016). The Durban Conference is thus remembered not only for the publicly pronounced antics of AIDS denialism of the former South African state president Thabo Mbeki but, more importantly, for the manner in which generalized AIDS treatment was put on the global agenda. This led to a "paradigm shift [for] ... thinking about global access issues" (Gregg Gonsalves of Gay Men's Health Crisis in New York, in Knight, 2006) and issues of activism to generalized access to ART spread from the South to parts of the North.

HIV and AIDS' visibility grew in stature. The allure to be part of the global movement fighting for access to ART in the global South grew apace. Programs such as the Global Media AIDS Initiative (GMAI), launched by Kofi Annan in 2004, emphasized the importance of the global media in responding to the disease, and its important function of raising awareness and breaking down stigma. Buy-in was attested as 20 media corporations representing 13 countries attended the GMAI launch where Bill Gates was the keynote speaker. Bill Roedy, who was the Vice-Chair of MTV Networks and the UNAIDS Goodwill Ambassador, was elected as GMAI's first Chair of the Leadership Committee. Accepting this accolade, he stated,

> If education is currently the only vaccine available to us, then the global media industry has in its hands the means to deliver that vaccine.
>
> (Roedy, 2004, in Knight, 2006)

The famous 46664 concerts, in association with MTV's "Staying Alive" campaign, were organized to raise awareness of HIV and AIDS globally. These concerts were called "46664" as remembrance of Nelson Mandela's prison number during his incarceration at Robben Island. The concerts not only attracted the rich and famous of the global North but appealed to increased support. The first HIV and AIDS concert was hosted in Cape Town, South Africa – the country in the world with the highest number of infected individuals. This first concert was followed by a concert in 2004 in Johannesburg and in 2005 in George, South Africa. The same year witnessed two other concerts – one in Madrid, Spain and one in Tromso, Norway. The appeal of these concerts was increased by the participation of an illustrious group of artists from all parts of the world. The late Joe Strummer, together with Bono of U2, wrote a special song for Nelson Mandela called "46664" in honor of this event.

This period from the early 2000s onward witnessed an unprecedented rise in prominence of HIV and AIDS. This surge in interest and commitment was not only limited to the political and economic domains but increasingly started shaping the AIDS cause as an appealing commodity that famous people wanted to be part of. After years of struggle and strife for recognition, the glory days for AIDS were finally arriving.

The fat years of funding

The World Bank initially cut its HIV and AIDS spending (falling from US$67 million in 1994 to US$41.7 million in 1997) but started realizing that previous developmental efforts – those that had taken place over the past 20–30 years – would be seriously jeopardized if assistance was not to be increased. The World Bank was thus the first organization to create a dedicated funding mechanism in light of HIV and AIDS as it approved its Multi-Country HIV and AIDS Program for Africa (MAP) in 2000. At first, a sum of US$500 million was authorized with another half a billion US dollars promised as and when the need arouse (Knight, 2006). Not only the influx of money but negotiations related to drug pricing and the Doha Declaration on TRIPS[4] and public health (in 2001) paved the way to offer more affordable ART to those countries with restricted resources and a growing ART demand.

The year 2001 also heralded the first talks and meetings that would lead to the creation of the Global Fund as political and financial commitment was gaining ground. During these deliberations, it was agreed that this fund would be targeting not only HIV and AIDS but also tuberculosis (TB) and malaria. Not only foreign aid but also internal prioritization in terms of budgeting was secured by African leaders at the Organization for African Unity summit in 2001. African leaders pledged a contribution of 15% of their national budgets to improve healthcare in general. There was also consensus that HIV and AIDS posed a massive threat to their countries' health and well-being. It was at this occasion when Kofi Annan proposed his idea of a "war chest" of money to combat the scourge, calling for contributions from developing and developed countries of roughly US$7 billion to US$10 billion every year for a protracted period. Soon after this invitation, US President George W Bush pledged US$200 million to complement Annan's vision. France and the UK followed suit with contributions of US$300 and Kofi Annan himself donated US$100,000 from a prize he had received. This contribution was matched by the International Olympic Committee, and the Bill & Melinda Gates Foundation also bequeathed US$100 million to the fledgling fund (Knight, 2006). This fund then started disbursing international donations in 2002 to subsidize ART in countries hard hit and unable to afford generalized ART. The functioning of the Global Fund also positioned a new funding model that aimed toward reconciling requests for funding with actual strategic processes of those countries where the requests emanated from. These requests had, however, to be in line with the strategic choices set out by the Global Fund itself in order to maximize the impact of spending of its scarce resources (Cohen & Guthrie, 2014).

The Global Fund's main collaborators are governments, civil society, the private sector, and communities that are affected by this triumvirate of scourges that the Fund set out to combat. In order to supplement existing initiatives, the Fund also collaborates with other bilateral and multilateral organizations already active in the field. No less than US$15.6 billion had been approved through Global Health channeling since it first started operating, and 57% of the fund's money has been dispensed in sub-Saharan Africa. Nevertheless, the Global Fund was not to be the sole heavyweight of financial assistance in the fight against HIV and AIDS. A rather surprising turn of events was the announcement in 2003 during the State of the Union Address of the then US President George W. Bush. He announced the President's Emergency Plan for AIDS Relief (referred to as PEPFAR). PEPFAR would allocate US$15 billion over five years (2003–2008) to respond to HIV and AIDS in those countries hardest hit by the scourge, notably in Africa. In July 2008, PEPFAR was reauthorized with an even more impressive dedicated contribution of US$ 48 billion approved for the 2009–2013 financial years.

Speculative accounts as to the founding of PEPFAR include an array of assumptions. First related to notions of securitization, this generous offer was seen in light of generalized American fears of terrorism in destabilized contexts brought about by HIV and AIDS and in the wake of 9/11. Second, it is even postulated that President Bush's overt evangelical Christian beliefs – firmly rooted in altruism and charity – were the root cause for such benevolent actions. A third hypothesis, more cynical, is that this announcement could have been used in an attempt to mitigate the announcement of his intention to start war in Iraq, which was announced in the same speech (Behrman, 2004). Another indication as to the rationale behind this gesture of largess is noted in Knight's (2006) account of the first ten years of UNAIDS. In this meticulous rendition of UNAIDS' activities and access to inside information perhaps unknown to the general public, she refers to a 2002 briefing note to Peter Piot that indicated that the White House seriously considered increasing its spending on HIV after the perusal of the unpublished UNAIDS analysis document that explained optimal spending allocations among major global donors. Packard (2016) states that the creation of this bilateral program for AIDS was a reflection of the ongoing concerns about the ineffectiveness of multilateral organizations (such as the Global Fund). It was also assumed that PEPFAR could respond more effectively to the USA's economic and strategic interests in those areas where their aid would be effective. Protecting their interests included protective measures such as disallowing the financing of generic drugs (and thereby benefitting US pharmaceutical companies). This precondition was, however, after intense activist objections, revoked.

Whatever the reason or combination of reasons behind the creation of PEPFAR, it does represent the world's largest international health program, and the American government has thus contributed the highest sum of money toward a single disease in the history of humankind. This obviously has entailed an unparalleled involvement in African health by the USA and its affiliate institutions.

There has been a range of controversies surrounding PEPFAR's policies and the preconditions governing the disbursements of funds. Their initial focus mainly on prevention has led to indignation from a chorus of international voices. For example, it was stipulated that at least one-third of the prevention funds be earmarked for abstinence programs and church-based interventions were not to distribute condoms (Packard, 2016). This corresponds sharply to the continuing moral overtones that HIV and AIDS has given rise to throughout its historic unfolding. Moreover, it has been shown that of the 61 million people served by the PEPFAR sponsored interventions between 2004 and 2007, 40 million of these people were in programs only promoting abstinence and/or being faithful (the "A" and "B" of the ABC of prevention – dropping the "C" which means to "condomize"). Shockingly, given the amount of money at stake, it was found that these intervention programs had ultimately no impact on affecting the prevention of new HIV infections in Africa (McNeil, 2015b). By law, US government funding cannot be used for harm reduction programs either, such as needle exchange for injecting drug users. However, given its sheer financial commitment and investment, and the strictness associated with implementation and choice of programs, PEPFAR has been influential in shaping a new context of development and philanthropic aid, largely determined by global public health dictates (Oomman et al., 2007). The start of Africa's ART era, a period of new hope and survival captured in incredible tales of resurrection and a new lease on life, was ushered in largely by the contributions made available through the Global Fund and PEPFAR.

As indicated in Chapter 1, the global response, especially the unprecedented allocation of monetary resources, has been severely criticized from various sources as wasteful and ineffective. However, the UN agency still maintains that ramping up the HIV response, as suggested by the UNAIDS (2014b) report titled *Fast-Track. Ending the AIDS Epidemic by 2030*, could amount to a 17-fold return on countries' investments in the fight. This report, in a dramatic and visually striking manner, simultaneously celebrates and cautions, by boldly stating,

> We have bent the trajectory of the AIDS epidemic.
>   Now we have five years.
>   To break the epidemic.
>   Or we risk the epidemic springing back even stronger.
>
> (UNAIDS, 2014b)

It is true that the global response to HIV and AIDS at the dawn of the treatment era has been unparalleled. According to UNAIDS, between 2007 and 2008, global funding expanded from US$11.3 billion to US$13.7 billion, and in the period between 2001 and 2009, funding for the fight against HIV increased almost ninefold (Deghaye & Whiteside, 2012). However, the reality today is that funding is flat-lining or decreasing altogether. Are we risking the epidemic to spring back even stronger? Another distressing critique leveled at PEPFAR and other US bilateral programs is the considerate amounts of donor funding that goes toward overhead expenses, equipment, traveling, salary, and benefit packages for staff from the USA who are tasked with evaluation and other related activities in areas where the funding is disbursed (Redfield, 2012). The increase in critical studies of foreign aid that explains instances of collateral damage or a seemingly benign, legitimate siphoning off of money, leads to cynicism and suspicion as to the true effects and intentions of these programs.

And then ... the lean years of funding

The 2008 global financial crisis, ongoing fiscal constraints, and unprecedented crises within the global North all presage a global shift in the definition of "crises." In 2015, it was announced that the Millennium Development Goal 6 – that aimed toward halting and reversing the spread of HIV – was reached, as well as the target of getting 15 million people on treatment by 2015 – an objective that was met nine months prior to the set deadline (UNAIDS, 2015b). In 2014, it was estimated that of the 14.9 million people receiving ART globally, 13.5 million of these lived in low- and middle-income countries (WHO, 2015a). Despite celebrations and positive news, new infections are not abating and new guidelines from WHO state that ART will have the most significant impact if started immediately after a person is diagnosed with HIV. This increased, vigorous roll-out, together with sustaining those already on treatment, and the increasing promises of PrEP all lead to the agonizing question: where will the money come from?

The heavyweights are slowly but surely moving out and moving on. The second phase of PEPFAR (2009–2014) coincided with the global economic crisis as well as with political transition within the USA. The US government funding for ART through PEPFAR flat-lined and declined 10% between 2009 and 2010 (Kates et al., 2011). It is said that the Obama administration's Global Health Initiative shifted its focus toward maternal and child health (Sahoo, 2010) despite its extending PEPFAR's budget to US$51 billion over six years. Critics have pointed out that this sum was not in line with the US$48 billion that former president Obama pledged to be rolled out from 2013, or the added US$1 billion increase per year that he promised during his election campaign. It is estimated that this collapse in funding would lead to 1 million people not receiving ART, as well as to 2.9 million women not receiving prevention-of-mother-to-child-transmission (PMTCT) interventions (ICASO, 2015). Former president Obama defended this change in funding by stating that PEPFAR would be cooperating with multilateral organizations (like the Global Fund and UNAIDS) and would be effecting bilateral programs to be more integrated in its approach to fight a variety of diseases. It was also said that the aim would be to increasingly focus on improving overall health and, therefore, to strengthen health systems, thereby echoing the "discourse of sustainability" (Ingram, 2013).

As for the global financial scene, fiscal austerity ushered in a series of new reforms with the aim of transforming PEPFAR programs and other initiatives away from an emergency response vested in exceptionalism, to a more sustainable model, strongly contingent upon monitoring and evaluation, implementation science, and evidence-based results. A strong focus on collaboration with recipient governments in the name of sustainability also ensued. This shift in focus emerged not only because of fiscal constraints but also because it was increasingly acknowledged that the first phase of PEPFAR interventions was too focused on achieving impressive targets at the expense of recording actual measurable effects. This scathing critique was instrumental in shifting US government funding (including PEPFAR) to interventions with concrete, measurable impacts, translated into so-called sustainable interventions.

Overall, global health growth in terms of global health funding staggered to a mere 4%, falling to no growth at all in 2010 and 2011 (Garrett, 2012). The US and other donations to the Global Fund have declined, and this has led to the Fund being forced to renegotiate some of its previous plans. All plans approved for funding in Round 8 were to be decreased by 10%. The ninth round of funding was to be deferred by six months and was the only round to take place during 2009. The second phase of Global Fund donations had to contend with a 25% cut in existing and future grants. In an interview with the Head of the Global Fund in 2009, Michel Kazatchkine, he openly acknowledged that the demand for funds in 2009 had exceeded the supply, and that this happened for the first time in the existence of the Global Fund. He also announced the suspension of 2010 funding to 2011 in order to replenish funds. When 2011 arrived, the Global Fund was in no position to continue with another round of funding and subsequently had to cancel Round 11, because of donors not owning up to their commitments.

UNAIDS then estimated that by 2015, US$24 billion would have been needed for a comprehensive HIV and AIDS response, but that only US$17 billion would have been forthcoming. New pledges do not remotely add up to the necessary budget. It was also predicted that financial needs related to HIV and AIDS interventions would increase until at least 2020 (Whiteside & Strauss, 2014).

These global financial vicissitudes obviously had a major negative effect on African countries hugely dependent and reliant on donor assistance. Although both donor leaders (PEPFAR and the Global Fund) have committed to sustain existing funding to ART programs, the future of expanded treatment is looking increasingly bleak and uncertain. This has led to some arguing that the "golden age" of global health funding, firmly rooted in AIDS exceptionalism, was dealt a deathblow (Rushton & Williams, 2011; Ingram, 2013). Economists are now pointing to the fact that the "best choices when resources are scarce" principle was not upheld during the "emergency era" of HIV and AIDS funding. This was greatly attributed to poor donor coordination, funds that were not budgeted for, and the fact that governments were not encouraged to provide these funds systematically. In addition, the resources were spread thinly to achieve as much impact with limited means (Deghaye & Whiteside, 2012). The pendulum is starting to swing toward the opposite extreme as we face the tightening of donor taps and witness increased emphasis on "strategic investment" that increasingly directs resources to areas where the greatest impact will be felt and to ensure the greatest value for money. Empirical evidence as to the greatest investment success stories is becoming the new norm, as could be concluded by the "joke" of Patrick Gaspard, the US Ambassador in South Africa, during his plenary address at the 7th South African AIDS Conference in 2015,

In God we trust, but everyone else, bring the data!

This shift in emphasis now steers toward a new obsession of measured and evidence-based cost-effective interventions. This new fixation greatly revolves around the push for new technical solutions, such as medically performed male circumcision, treatment as prevention (TasP), PrEP, new ART formulations, and the rationalization of procurement, logistics, and supply chain management. These cost-effective and "proven" initiatives will be the darlings of donor programs in years to come. Initially, the HIV and AIDS response was characterized by its rather contradictory manifestation. First, of resisting neoliberal abandonment as witnessed in the 1980s and 1990s, especially with the imposition of the much loathed structural adjustment programs that led to a great deal of destruction on the African continent. Second, the initial HIV and AIDS response also paved the way for "neoliberal developmentalism" with its preoccupation of saving lives together with the forging of new partnership, engendering empowerment, exercising leverage, and supporting unprecedented advocacy (Ingram, 2013).

The initial response to HIV and AIDS, when the epidemic first appeared to hold a real global threat, was thus marred by initial reluctance, divided loyalties, scathing stereotypes, a lack of leadership, and selfish pursuit of vested interests. For too long, the focus was more on securing legitimacy and, therefore, power and not on the actual unfolding of the scourge. In a rather damning opinion of the UN's initial response to HIV and AIDS, Stephen Lewis, who was the former Special Envoy of the UN Secretary-General for HIV and AIDS in Africa, had the following to say,

> I think that the absence of leadership, which UNAIDS could not overcome, at the center of the UN system has resulted in far less progress than should otherwise have been the case. There is no question in my mind that, when history is written, when the significant history of the pandemic is written, the inability of the UN to orchestrate a response far more vigorous, far more effective, far more searching than the response we've had thus far, that that will be seen as one of the sad components of the pandemic. That is not – I don't really believe that's a commentary on UNAIDS. I think it goes much further than that; I think it goes to the heads of agencies and to the Heads of the [UN] Secretariat.
>
> (Lewis in Knight, 2006)

Whereas the HIV and AIDS epidemic was at the root of expanded global health funding and interventions as from the 1990s (albeit lethargic and uncoordinated as was just indicated), the spectacular development of new drugs boosted global health funding to unprecedented levels – thereby ushering in the era of normalization through biomedicalization (Packard, 2016).

The story of ART

History has taught us that the construction and subsequent implementation of knowledge, and the emergence of "revised" versions of knowledge, can have severe repercussions for some people. The story of HIV and its treatment are rife with examples of "changing discourses" – meticulously depicted mostly by social scientists – renditions that bear witness to the follies of science. After the initial euphoria of finding an effective treatment for HIV and AIDS, attention shifted to the pressing problem of treating people beyond the borders of the global North. In fact, it became increasingly evident that the HIV epidemic was expanding in areas far from North America and that it was manifesting in ways unrelated to developed world patterns.

The stark differences between the AIDS in industrialized, wealthy countries and the AIDS of African and other developing countries became glaringly evident at the 1996 International AIDS Conference in Vancouver, Canada, where the announcement of the effectiveness of highly active antiretroviral therapy (HAART) was first made. With its ironic conference slogan "One World, One Hope," and the majority of delegates and activists hailing from the global North, the protracted struggle for this expensive lifesaving treatment began for those – unable to afford it – all over the world. It was nothing more than a pipe dream for the vast majority of people in the developing world to access this elixir. At that point in time, one year's treatment would have cost around US$20,000 which made it wholly inaccessible to the majority of HIV-infected individuals. This also introduced the start of dramatic activism that would continue at future AIDS Conferences. This vocal activism acted (as it still does) to perform stimulating and uncomfortable moments of reflection within these rational and orderly academic and biomedical conferences. At the conference in 1996, activists theatrically threw fake money, printed with the names of "Big Pharma" on stages where presenters were seated to labor the point that HAART prices had to be reduced (Knight, 2006).

It was the French president of the time, Jacques Chirac, who first called for an international fund to provide ART to all countries in need thereof. He made this announcement at the ICASA meeting in Abidjan in the Ivory Coast in December 1997, just over one year after the watershed Vancouver Conference. His suggestion was, however, dismissed by fellow donors based on fears related to sustainability and feasibility in countries with weak health systems. Underdevelopment, in the areas where HIV and AIDS started making a noticeable impact, was put forward as a major obstacle to roll out ART in contexts other than the global North. Incredible public pronouncements were uttered about these hard-hit areas and their inhabitants where AIDS was increasingly taking its toll, and this discourse largely deferred the possibility of making ART available to HIV-positive Africans. According to Andrew Natsios, who then headed the US Agency for International Development under the Bush administration, the problem with extending ART to Africans lay with the people in Africa themselves who

> don't know what Western time is. You have to take these [AIDS] drugs a certain number of hours each day, or they don't work. Many people in Africa have never seen a clock or a watch their entire lives. And if you say, one o'clock in the afternoon, they do not know what you are talking about. They know morning, they know noon, they know evening, they know the darkness at night.
>
> (Herbert, 2001)

This purported African ignorance and other stereotypical ideas related to uncivil and chaotic circumstances in Africa, together with the continent's weak health systems, therefore, conjured up images of the potential apocalyptic treatment-resistant strains as the only outcome of ART access in Africa. This led to the widespread and justified reluctance to disperse ART to underdeveloped regions. These places, mainly in Africa and particularly sub-Saharan Africa, were called places of "antiretroviral anarchy" and a "petri dish" for the creation of new treatment-resistant strains of HIV (Harries et al., 2001;

Popp & Fisher, 2002). Even the World Bank expressed caution, alleging that "problems with patient compliance are likely to be worse in low-income countries due to low education and the many other problems that poor people in developing countries face" (World Bank, 1999). The initial reason for international aid to extend their reach into these perceived backward areas – although initially by not providing ART – primarily revolved around perceived security threats that HIV posed.

Despite its initial reluctance, UNAIDS eventually attempted a pilot project dubbed the Drug Access Initiative, to provide the AIDS community with empirical data as to the feasibility of ART roll-out in the developing world. This pilot project involved four countries: Chile, Ivory Coast, Uganda, and Vietnam. After intense negotiations and ambiguous feelings, a list of conditions was drawn up and pharmaceutical companies agreed to provide ART at subsidized prices to those countries participating in this study. The prices would be reduced by approximately 40% of the developed world price, which stood at US$10,000 to US$12,000 per person annually. UNAIDS from their side, worked with the local healthcare infrastructures to ensure that the drugs would be distributed effectively and that the pharmaceutical companies' preoccupations – largely vested in concerns over corruption and intellectual property issues – were known and respected (Knight, 2006). The Drug Access Initiative signaled a breakthrough in terms of differential pricing for medicines from "big Pharma" given that there were still few generic suppliers of ART. However, toward 1999, increasing amounts of generic drugs started entering the market and soon gained legitimacy in a very protective and suspicious industry. Pressure, however, on pharmaceutical companies was mounting to increase treatment access to the developing world.[5] In May 2000, the Accelerating Access Initiative (AAI) was declared after a rather candid speech by WHO's Director-General, Gro Harlem Brundtland, who said,

> … squarely put, the drugs are in the North and the disease is in the South. This kind of inequity cannot continue … I wish to invite the pharmaceutical industry to join us now in taking a fresh and constructive look at how we can considerably increase access to relevant drugs.
>
> (Brundtland, 2000, in Knight, 2006)

Thus, the negotiations between UNAIDS and the pharmaceutical companies proceeded in order to explore the potential of accelerated and improved ART provisioning. Unfortunately, some African leaders saw these negotiations as dealings to which they were not invited and which consequently undermined their sovereignty. They, therefore, rebuffed these seemingly benevolent deeds. This grievance or misunderstanding (depending on the perspective on the matter) stands in contrast to the much-vaunted "definition" of global health referred to earlier, coined under dubious circumstances that undermined true global representation. Nevertheless, in the throes of this dispute, victory yet again outshone dissent, and the AAI negotiations managed to substantially reduce the prices of first-line ART to a cost of approximately US$1,200 per person per year. Consequently, after a number of successful treatment programs among HIV-positive people in Africa and elsewhere, mainly driven by the international organization *Médecins Sans Frontières*, the discourse started shifting rather dramatically. Underdevelopment, access to great numbers of "treatment naïve" populations, and desperate states with weak health systems turned into a "medical technologies market opportunity" (Crane, 2013). Today, international HIV research and global health programs increasingly covet diseased bodies in the underdeveloped world. This happens by way of "academic global health" which serves the purpose of (especially) US-based universities, to fulfill criteria of modules associated with "global health" where US students spend time in resource-poor, often African settings to witness, first-hand the suffering and shortcomings of these contexts and the consequences of the generalized lack of health commodities. The very conditions that once rendered ART roll-out unimaginable started attracting growing global interest, turning this state of affairs in the developing world into what Crane (2013) terms "valuable inequalities."

Another global force that had to be reckoned with was the extraordinary and robust civic voice that grew in stature in demanding access to lifesaving treatment. Activists were, and continue to be, the biggest ally of affordable and accessible ART in the world. Unparalleled global solidarity grew out of the race for ART, especially its universal availability in all countries where people faced HIV infected. This led to spirited demonstrations at the International AIDS Conference in Durban in 2000, and increasing calls on the provision of cheaper, generic versions of unaffordable drugs. The US-based activist group, Act Up, fired up a persistent campaign against the US government for its support to pharmaceutical companies' protective patent legislation (Smith & Whiteside, 2010). Despite the misgivings of the powerful pharmaceutical industry, low- to middle-income countries, such as Brazil, India, and South Africa, started manufacturing, exporting, and/or importing generic ART for domestic use (Grady, 2001). In 1997, a consortium of 40 pharmaceutical companies filed a lawsuit against Nelson Mandela's South African Government against legislation that would enable the production and/or importation of generic medical treatments. This lawsuit was eventually dropped as the Clinton Administration withdrew support for the pharmaceuticals' cause, following intense picketing by activists during Al Gore's Presidential Campaign with catchy slogans such as "Gore's Greed Kills" (Cooper et al., 2001). The eventual amendment of the TRIPS agreement from the World Trade Organization (WTO), known as the Doha Declaration (as discussed earlier), made it possible for countries facing terrible scourges, such as HIV and AIDS, to revert to emergency measures, including the production and/or importation of generic medicines, in order to maintain their public health and, therefore, also the global public health.[6]

Equally extraordinary was the 2002 landmark Constitutional Court ruling in South Africa which compelled the South African state to implement a program of universal coverage of mother-to-child transmission of HIV and AIDS, also known as PMTCT (Heywood, 2003). The reverberating success of this litigation paved the way for continued activism to universal ART coverage.

The immediate future of ART was writ large: the potent combination of activism in the name of universal human rights, humanitarianism, and the unprecedented scientific opportunities that HIV and AIDS and its treatment offered, became increasingly evident to politicians, academics, activists, and people living with HIV and AIDS (PLWHAs). Unparalleled funding programs, as earlier discussed, saw the light and were greatly responsible for the massive scale-up of ART access globally. Today, however, the future of ART is less clear. In a time of austerity and increased rationalization, and by framing the continued and sustained access to ART as a "ballooning entitlement burden" (Over, 2008) instead of as a right or a humanitarian security necessity, we are finding ourselves in an insecure futurity as to the quandary of sustainable ART access. Despite this looming tragedy related to funding and sustained ART programs, in June 2009, UNAIDS and the World Bank released a report to preempt and to prepare for the onslaught in donor funding cuts (UNAIDS & World Bank, 2009). The report acknowledged that the consequences would be dire: increased mortality and morbidity, unforeseen interruptions and inability to extend treatment, increased risk of HIV transmission, higher future financial expenditures, and increased burdens on already troubled health systems. In short, the report warned of the reversal of years of work and funding related to economic and social development advances. This report continues to make several concrete suggestions to mitigate these adverse effects. Organizations, such as ARV Access for Africa (AA4A), are instrumental in responding to ART-related problems, such as stock-outs, and serve as a provider of "emergency ARVs" that could be mobilized within 24 hours to reach 80% of sub-Saharan destinations within one week. There have also been increased calls on governments to strengthen program efficiency and cost-effectiveness. Streamlining programs and focusing on interventions with a good record of accomplishment of evidence-based results are also said to be prioritized (UNAIDS & World Bank, 2009).

There is thus no room for complacency in the current ART climate. The continued availability of these wonder pills should not be taken for granted. In addition, not all ART is the same. In fact, the technology related to the micro workings of these drugs and pharmacogenetics are constantly evolving, and yet again, unequally so between the haves and the have-nots of our unequal global village. Issues pertaining to the quality of drugs, drug quantities, or the known side effects of certain treatment options, and drug resistance that will require second- and third-line regimes are all part of the continued struggle for treatment, and where developing countries could also become a dumping ground for excess, obsolete treatment regimens.

South Africa in a time of "AIDS Acceptance"[7]

> South Africa has one of the highest national investments in AIDS in the world. We must continue to work together in the next five years to ensure that South Africa and its partners continue to invest in the national response so that we stay ahead of the AIDS epidemic here.
>
> (Michel Sidibé, UNAIDS Executive Director; UNAIDS, 2015a)

South Africa has traced an interesting history in the chronicles of the AIDS epidemic. The tragic coincidence between the end of apartheid and the emergence of a serious AIDS epidemic, as already highlighted, was an historical confluence almost too cruel to contemplate. Nevertheless, the entrenched vestiges of apartheid – intended and unintended – together with newfound freedom, invoked an intersectionality of circumstances that would catapult this dreaded disease into the global realm of exceptionality. These exceptional circumstances were probably the reason why so many people, especially academics from all corners of the earth, were tolerant and understanding of the infamous era of AIDS denialism. There were, however, calls to put former president Thabo Mbeki – the main voice behind the denialist saga – on trial for genocide given his sustained refusal to implement any form of ART program within the borders of South Africa. This dark patch in the history of AIDS in South Africa was to be analyzed and explained, and its brutality and blatancy somehow made the South African epidemic even more exotic to study. In tandem with ensuing episodes emphasizing AIDS denialism and the search to find an "African cure for an African illness" (Geffen, 2010), an exceptional activist movement – with its objectives firmly rooted in individual and communal rights for people with HIV and reminiscent of anti-apartheid advocacy – was gaining strength. Despite the short-lived euphoria of a united front (between the state and activists) against the pharmaceutical companies that dragged the South African government to court over its Medicine and Related Substances Act, the HIV and AIDS field was soon to be characterized by intense contestation between government and civil society (Schneider, 2002; Butler, 2005; Mbali, 2005). This led to what London and Schneider (2012) call

> a discourse saturated in "rights talk" on all sides: on the one hand, the right to individual autonomy, access to treatment and a "scientific" approach to HIV/AIDS drawing on constitutional notions of individual human rights; on the other hand, appeals to different kinds of entitlements – national sovereignty, unique African responses, cultural dignity and communal rights.

Ironically, the discourse of each of these camps (activists *vs.* dissidents) claimed the representation of the plight of the many poor, affected South African citizens and therefore drew on "deeply held collective experiences"

(London & Schneider, 2012). These experiences were related to the recent struggle against apartheid and its abuses of individual freedoms (discourses from the activist cohort), on the one side, and of colonialism, apartheid, and Western hegemony (discourses from the state, personified by Mbeki during his free-reign interpretation of HIV and AIDS), on the other. Despite its morbid ramifications, South Africa's HIV epidemic and the denialist phase thus provided a fruitful opportunity to contemplate the post-apartheid South African society, past and present, and has yielded an astonishing and unprecedented array of initiatives ranging from scientific enquiries, policy formulation, virulent activism, and newly shaped subjectivities (Fassin, 2007).

However, the interests have shifted, and we are currently finding ourselves squarely in an era marked by technocratic and biomedical approaches to treatments and large-scale normalization. South Africa is managing the world's largest ART program, and in this context, Navario et al. (2012) mention a sobering fact,

> It is axiomatic that the battle against HIV/AIDS globally will not be won if success is not achieved within South Africa, which hosts 20 per cent of the world's people living with HIV/AIDS.

HIV being in its fourth decade as a known and researched disease, the focus is now to apply all energies to eradicate the scourge and to prevent its continued renewal and manifestation in bodies. Strange ideas have been invoked to end HIV: programs enticing abstinence from sex, and the range of practices and ideas clustered under the aforementioned "AIDS denialism," are probably the most bizarre manifestations of trying to "end" HIV and AIDS (or in the case of AIDS denialism, to disregard it in its entirety and to view it rather as a major conspiracy against Africans and African culture). Contemporary South Africa is, however – like the rest of the world – increasingly conventional in fighting the disease, even exceptionally so.

Dramatically depicted in the documentary of the Treatment Action Campaign (TAC), *Taking HAART*, the number of people on ART compared to the number of infections due to AIDS and related deaths is visually evidenced in the massive surge of South Africans who have access to lifesaving drugs. After access, the major issues of expanding and sustaining ART are now of paramount importance. In an era of "AIDS Acceptance" and the accompanying political will, fiscal considerations constitute a major potential impediment to guarantee this sustainable access to ART. However, critically engaging with issues of normalization is also a process that should not fall by the wayside in a climate of strict biomedical interventions.

At the South African AIDS Conference in June 2015, the then Deputy-President Cyril Ramaphosa (who has since become South Africa's president) proudly stated that the South African government is responsible for more than 80% of HIV and AIDS and TB funding, although he did caution that treatment roll-out cannot continue unabatedly.[8] During his address at this illustrious gathering, he stated the sobering fact that "putting more people on treatment is not sustainable; we have to stop new infections."

With the world's largest number of HIV-positive people and one of the greatest ART programs in the world, South Africa yet again takes its seat in the category of exceptionalism. In fact, as indicated by the earlier quote of Navario et al. (2012), the onus of eradicating HIV and AIDS (in the global South where infections are still prevalent) rests largely on the successes of the South African HIV program. Looking at the numbers more intently, it shows that external aid, according to estimates of the South African Treasury, amounts to R5 billion to R6 billion a year. This indicates that South Africa is also largely dependent on the charity and largess of the global North, and our successes in relation to ART will, therefore, also be at the mercy of this "mobile sovereignty" (Pandolfi, 2000). South Africa can then be added to the following definition of arbitrariness, uttered by Bernard Schwartlander of the UNAIDS,

> The lives of more than 80 per cent of the people who receive AIDS treatment in Africa depend every morning on whether or not a donor writes another cheque.
>
> (In IRIN, 2012)

And despite Ramaphosa's forewarnings, the new WHO guidelines recommend that people be initiated onto ART as soon as their seropositive status is ascertained, and this new policy direction is followed by the South African government in their current AIDS policy.[9] Early treatment initiation has been the recent fine-tuning of the "magic bullet" recipe of ART as it would potentially lead to better health outcomes, as well as to averting new infections, which remains a huge hurdle in the South African fight against HIV, especially among young women. Early treatment initiation, together with the promises of the current roll-out of PrEP, and other indirect costs associated with HIV are all slowly depleting the South African budget in times of slow economic growth and where budgetary demands are certainly not decreasing.[10] In addition and as described earlier on, it is widely acknowledged that international donor aid, especially aimed at HIV and AIDS as such, is flat-lining and even decreasing. This is evident in the trends of external aid over the years: in 2009/2010, external aid added 16.4% to the South African government's fight against HIV and AIDS and TB. From 2007 to 2010, external sources rose significantly by 68% from R1.3 billion to R2.14 billion (Cohen & Guthrie, 2014). However, now we are witnessing a slow decrease of external funding where total funding for HIV and AIDS and TB from all external partners was projected to have decreased to R5 billion in 2015/2016 from R5.6 billion in 2012/2013 (Cohen & Guthrie, 2014). This slowdown can be attributed to the downturn of the global economy and to the increase of other pressing matters, such as new outbreaks of other diseases (the 2014 Ebola outbreak) and the unprecedented emergency migrations into Europe, which all contribute to a shift in priorities and, therefore, reductions in financial aid from external partners to address HIV and AIDS. Already in 2012, the US government announced that South Africa was to become the first country to "nationalize" its PEPFAR program by scaling down on funding and by handing back increased "responsibility" to the South African government to manage its HIV and AIDS programs (Govender, 2012).

South Africa's national strategic plans

Even when the South African government (personified by former Mbeki and his then Minister of Health, the late Manto Tsabalala-Msimang) was impetuously pursuing its alternative views of defining and treating HIV and AIDS, the Health Ministry still upheld a rather "conventional" National Strategic Plan of 2000–2005 (The Operational Plan for Comprehensive HIV and AIDS Care, Management, and Treatment). Earlier, the incumbent government (the ANC), together with the old regime (the Health Ministry of the National Party's government), and the United Democratic Front actually started responding to the disease as soon as in 1992 with the first meeting of the National AIDS Convention of South Africa (NACOSA). NACOSA was created to institute a robust and comprehensive national AIDS response as from 1994 (Butler, 2005). Despite its good intentions, the plan was insufficiently informed by the social and institutional realities that characterized the South African context (Butler, 2005). This initial HIV and AIDS governance was equally marred by accusations of financial mismanagement of the then Minister of Health, Dr Nkosazana Dlamini-Zuma, thereby paving the way for what would become the much-scrutinized era of "AIDS Denialism."

The National AIDS Plan (2000–2005) also did not consider the overall inability of the prevailing infrastructure and functional organizations to be accountable for the new criteria as set out by the Strategic Plan. In fact, it is considered that this policy led to an increase in fragmentations in healthcare. Local administrations were completely unable to orchestrate the functioning and troubleshooting that this National AIDS Plan required (Schneider & Stein, 2001). Tragically, this led to the inability of the National AIDS Plan to delay the transmission of HIV and AIDS, and neither could the National AIDS Plan provide ART to those in urgent need thereof. A reformulation of this Plan led to the conception of a new Plan (2007–2011) which was welcomed as the most dynamic and comprehensive document yet on AIDS issues within South Africa (Wouters et al., 2010). For the first time, not only national but also nongovernmental and civil bodies were incorporated into its planning and execution. This Plan strongly prioritized prevention, especially PMTCT as well as other forms of prevention, focusing on the youth. More importantly, it also announced the roll-out of ART and included the important areas of HIV research and monitoring and surveillance of HIV activities (Wouters et al., 2010). It is rather unsurprising that this Plan could not deliver on all its intended ambitious goals. The same issues prevailed, such as poor planning, poor budgeting, and structural realities, especially related to the pernicious problem of limited human resources for health.[11] This then unfortunately led to limited successes to expand ART to the majority of PLWHAs. In general, the intended projections set out in the Plan and the realities linked to concrete implementation, simply did not converge.

The subsequent Strategic Plan's (2011–2016) cost was estimated to be around R133.5 billion for the five-year period. It is indicated that the 2013/2014 annual cost of the stipulated response is R24 billion and that this amount would be rising to R32.6 billion for the year 2016/2017. During this period, the ambitious plan was introduced to increase the number of those who are on ART – from 1.9 million (at the end of 2012) to approximately 4.2 million over a five-year period. Also included in this new Plan was to screen 15–25 million people per year for HIV and TB, to carry out 4.3 million medical male circumcisions, and to treat 400,000 adults per year for pulmonary TB.

It has been noted by Cohen and Guthrie (2014) that HIV and TB testing and treatment include no less than 85% of the total cost of the response. This is largely due to the ambitious treatment targets that the Plan set out to achieve and its accumulative costs. However, more alarmingly, this large allocation to one aspect of the HIV and TB response is linked to the fact that the costs of other nonbiomedical programs were underestimated, because of a lack of costing evidence at the time of budgeting. The programs not included in the initial cost prediction for the NSP were identified by Cohen and Guthrie (2014) as being programs related to: "substance abuse, gender-based violence, migrations, social mobilization, community systems strengthening, certain key populations and research."

In addition, the annual financial shortfall between the available resources *vis-à-vis* actual requirements was estimated to have increased from R2.6 billion to R5 billion from 2014 to 2017 due to an increase in the scale of priority and the tightening of external sources of funding (Cohen & Guthrie, 2014). In fact, the South African government is increasingly faced with the predicament to carefully manage its spending priorities as the country is facing intensifying strike actions from a variety of sectors,[12] infrastructural collapse, and increasing bailouts from government to dysfunctional parastatals.

The "post-colonial paradox" in a time of HIV and AIDS: disequilibrium of priorities?

The South African government has been involved in intricate behind-the-scenes negotiations to see to the realization of one of the world's largest ART programs. They have, for example, managed to negotiate substantial decreases of the price for viral load testing as this testing is paramount in measuring the state of health of those who are HIV positive. This test is equally important for people who are on ART as it indicates the invisible progression or regression of the virus. The Health Department's ART tender processes have also managed to bring ART prices down considerably. In 2012, this negotiation led to a saving of no less than R4.7 billion (Deghaye & Whiteside, 2012).

Despite these cost-saving measures that were negotiated, South Africa's health budget has had to be cut substantially due to the global financial crisis. Perturbing estimated amounts are mentioned to mark the shortfall in the country's public sector ART program. It is also worrying that large private firms, especially mining companies, are probably going to tighten their HIV prevention programs, which will have an effect on many employees and their families. It is equally disturbing that the TAC, South Africa's best-known activist group, which also provides treatment, counseling, and HIV testing, is slowly losing its grip on securing adequate funding to proceed with its much-needed activities. The effect of less funding led to the closure of six of their provincial offices.

As for the global heavyweights, it is estimated that in 2015, the Global Fund and PEPFAR will cover 95% of Development Partner funding (Cohen & Guthrie, 2014). PEPFAR has provided nearly half of committed programmatic HIV financing in South Africa since 2004, and it is unlikely that this supply of funding will increase in the next few years due to opposing global health priorities and an overall tightening of budgets (Navario et al., 2012). In fact, PEPFAR has systematically been decreasing its annual financing in South Africa from an astounding R4.5 billion a couple of years ago to a projected stable investment of R2.25 billion per year in 2017 (Cohen & Guthrie, 2014). In addition to this shrinkage in funding, PEPFAR's focus has altered and now centers less on treatment and more on prevention and technical support. It is estimated that over 40% of their annual contribution will be spent on prevention interventions.

The Global Fund's contribution is seemingly more stable over the medium to long term with the caveat that the allocated grants perform acceptably. A dedicated funding stream for TB commenced in 2013/2014 and amounts to R180 million per annum. This initiative is also expected to remain rather stable over the medium to long term. Despite stability and slight decreases, some sub-programs are expected to have rather substantial financial shortfalls between supply and demand, and these sub-programs include ART, TB, and HCT. In 2012/2013 already, the estimated financial variance for ART was approximately R4.6 billion. The estimates for TB was near R1.4 billion, and for HCT, it was calculated to amount to roughly R1 billion. The ART sub-program displays the most virulent growth in the funding gap, because of the resources required to achieve the ambitious target coverage that has increased from 2.6 million individuals on treatment in 2012/2013 to 4.2 million people on ART by 2015/2016 (Cohen & Guthrie, 2014).

The flagship status of South Africa's HIV and AIDS and TB response, especially as it pertains to availability and access to ART, inevitably leads to the crowding out of investment in other health programs. It has been shown that the consolidated national and provincial HIV and AIDS distributions, proportionate to consolidated health expenditures, are expected to increase from 7.9% in 2012/2013 to 8.8% in 2013/2014. As for 2015/2016, this increase is estimated to grow by 10% notwithstanding the lack of growth in the financial distributions to health from the overall national budget. The national health budget has seen a decrease from 12% of the national budget in 2012/2013 to 11.4% in 2015/2016 (Cohen & Guthrie, 2014), and this, despite the well-acknowledged quadruple burden of disease that plagues South Africa. In addition, demands are only growing as WHO are recommending new guidelines for earlier treatment onset, and as we fail to prevent infections, especially among our young female population. This is all happening while the South African budget's general demands are swelling apace.

According international "flagship" status to South Africa's national HIV and AIDS response in relation to its ART program inevitably comes at a cost. The focus is narrowly set on treatment, inasmuch as the National Strategic Plan flagrantly omitted the budgetary requirements for a host of nonbiomedical costs directly related to the disease and to issues of (nonbiomedical) prevention. This is telling of the increased predominance of the pharmaceuticalization of HIV and the sole focus on treatment targets. There seems to be an increasing governmental commitment to ART, inevitably at the expense of other health issues, as can be witnessed by the overall budgetary cuts in the healthcare sector. In addition, HIV and concomitant HIV funding are prime examples of the maneuvering of global health activities where there is an interesting, yet troubling conjunction of humanitarian, charitable work, on the one hand, and geopolitical strategizing, vast scientific opportunity, and facile access to diseased bodies in quantities and qualities absent in the global North, on the other (Crane, 2013). Lakoff (2010) sees this conjunction of the "two regimes of global health" as less troubling and concludes that they should be understood as complementary,

> … humanitarian biomedicine could be seen as offering a philanthropic palliative to nation-states lacking public health infrastructure in exchange for the right of international health organizations to monitor their populations for outbreaks that might threaten wealthy nations.
>
> (Lakoff, 2010)

A narrow response to HIV and AIDS, focused solely on treatment, is a "safe" option as it rests upon tried and tested notions of saving lives. Contrarily, however, this overly simplified response in the current climate of global health happens to the detriment of more expansive or horizontal developmental targets that combine a host of issues. Of late, this tension has been present in the response from donors, like PEPFAR. This tension, according to Ingram (2013), reflects a "crucial fault line" in the response to HIV and AIDS in general. Does it represent an "exceptional humanitarian and security intervention premised upon a kind of bio-political minimalism ('saving lives'), or, a stepping stone towards a more radical, expansive and equitable global health agenda ('justice')"? Ingram continues to trace the relevance of this tension by stating that during the "phase of exceptionalism, securitization and scale-up, these propositions coexisted in an uneasy and largely unexamined symbiosis" (Ingram, 2013). And currently, with donor funding drying up and HIV becoming one disease among a host of others, these tensions are resurfacing again and should especially be worrying in the context of the South African HIV landscape where important future decisions are forged.

Notes

1 "International health," mainly spearheaded by WHO when it came into existence in 1948 during the Cold War period, had two main objectives: disease eradication and primary health care. Its focus was on collaboration between WHO and nation-states and national public health services. In contrast to its descendent "global health," international health functioned within the confines of state apparatuses (Lakoff, 2010).

2 The intricacies of the drama that unfolded in 2008 when Indonesia refused to provide WHO's Global Influenza Surveillance Network with virus strains of the H5N1 avian flu in order to develop more effective vaccines are telling of the politics of contemporary global health. This refusal was rooted in the sentiment that participation of "lesser" nations more than often do not translate into reciprocity when it comes to distributing the spoils of eventual results. A case in point is that affordability and access to vaccinations for dangerous new strands of influenza are often first available in rich, developed countries, despite the fact that these vaccines were developed because of the availability of strains to work with in the first place – strains emanating from countries that might need vaccination more urgently (see Lakoff, 2010).

3 "Development" is an intricate and contradictory process as was witnessed with the declaration of the "Development Decade" in the 1960s by J.F. Kennedy. He exhorted developing countries to increase their gross national product (GNP) by 5% from 1960 to 1970. This development decade saw substantial growth and GDP did rise, but somehow poverty persisted (see Packard, 2016).

4 The Doha Declaration in relation to the Trade-Related Aspects of Intellectual Property Rights or TRIPS agreement was an outcome of the Fourth World Trade Organization's Ministerial Conference that took place in Doha, Qatar. This declaration was "considered a key victory for developing and least developed countries, principally because it recognizes the countries' autonomy to implement the TRIPS Agreement in the best possible way for public health." The Doha Declaration emphasizes that TRIPS "can and should be interpreted and implemented in a manner supportive of WTO members' right to protect public health and, in particular, to promote access to medicines for all." The Declaration equally states that "public health crises, including those relating to HIV and AIDS, TB, malaria and other epidemics, can represent a national emergency" in which case governments can issue a compulsory license permitting, under specific circumstances, the utilization of patented products (in Knight, 2006). It has been argued that in South Africa, this opportunity has not been used to the full, given international (especially American) pressure. This restriction will be discussed in Chapter 4.

5 For example, the early 2000s witnessed the joint campaigns of TAC and international NGOs, such as *Médecins Sans Frontières*, Oxfam International, and Health-Gap that put the pharmaceutical industry under intense scrutiny. This eventually led to significant decreases in the pricing of ARV medicines (Heywood, 2009).

6 It is rather surprising that few governments have actually fully embraced this unique opportunity at maneuvering this amendment to suit their unique needs as can be witnessed with the criticism from the "Fix the Patents" campaign in

South Africa. London and Schneider also remark that few governments, in order to fulfill their human rights duties in relation to access to healthcare have actually wielded this powerful tool at their disposal (London & Schneider, 2012).

7 I use the term "AIDS Acceptance" as the contrary neologism of "AIDS Denialism."

8 It is anticipated that the total public HIV and AIDS allocation for the health sector would have increased sevenfold, from R2.1 billion in 2006/2007 to almost R15.3 billion in 2015/2016. This reflects the commitment that the South African government has made to the fight against HIV and AIDS and TB (Cohen & Guthrie, 2014).

9 At the International AIDS Conference in 2012, data from the HIV Prevention Trials Network (HPTN) 052 indicated that early ART initiation was very cost-effective. The analysis related to cost-effectiveness was modeled on South Africa and India. The HPTN 052 trial results were used to revise WHO's, which now recommend earlier initiation of ART, which will lead to "Treatment as Prevention."

10 In terms of balancing these various needs, Alice Decoteau (2013) refers to the "postcolonial paradox" which "entails a simultaneous need to respect the demands of neoliberal capital in order to compete successfully on the world market *and* a responsibility to redress entrenched inequality, secure legitimacy from the poor, and forge a national imaginary." This paradox is seen to be lived out daily in post-apartheid South Africa.

11 South Africa's healthcare system is characterized by persistent inequalities: the private sector, serving a minority of the South African population, hosts the large majority of healthcare professionals. The public sector, serving more than 80% of the South African population, faces a myriad of challenges related to resources, especially human resources, with a widely disparate distribution of healthcare workers. In addition, it was estimated that the ratio of nurses to patients within the public healthcare system as a whole dropped from 251 to 110 per 100,000 South Africans between 1994 and 2007 (Wouters et al., 2010).

12 As from 2015, strikes and demands from higher education students, (notably universities) for free tertiary education increased substantially combined with other demands that put increased pressure on the public coffer. These protests are equally indicative of a generalized movement to see more concrete transformations in these institutions. Other examples of unrelenting strike action are the crippling strikes in the mining sector that also led to the fatal shooting of miners by the police force in August 2012 that is sometimes referred to as "the Marikana massacre."

3 "Thin citizenship"[1] of community health workers

Introduction

Harnessing the expertise, time, and commitment of laypeople to advance developmental and healthcare is certainly not a new occurrence. It is, however, evident that the configuration of a variety of factors would dictate, to a large extent, the manner in which lay health work originates in the first place, as well as the manner in which it develops in specific contexts. The process of historicizing a phenomenon, in this case the extreme proliferation of lay and community health work in circumstances of escalating HIV infections and AIDS deaths, is valuable and insightful, but the history and contextualization thereof also implies a great deal of "irony and accident" (Mbembe, 2002) to fully grasp the minutiae of everyday life realities that come to shape this "parallel" or "informal" profession.

This chapter is focused on highlighting both historical contexts and the inevitable local translations and manifestations of community health work that give this informal cadre of healthcare work its unique character in an environment of high disease incidence and low levels of resources. It should be noted that the creation and the unparalleled spread of community health work, as it has taken shape as from the early 2000s within South Africa (but also elsewhere with high HIV prevalence in contexts of restrained resources and generalized precarity), was yet another unprecedented event brought about by the HIV and AIDS epidemic. This phenomenon, amply researched and scrutinized mostly in order to bring about proven beneficial and cost-effective interventions, is in itself undergoing a stage of normalization alongside the biomedicalization of HIV. In fact, in light of the increased demands on the healthcare sector with the increased availability of antiretroviral therapy (ART), it was estimated that the health workforce would have to be doubled every year between 2007 and 2017 to achieve the ambitious target of universal access (Barnighausen et al., 2007).[2] We will see that the South African government has responded to increasing the healthcare workforce by slowly and unpredictably incorporating community health workers (CHWs) into the official workings of the health system. But as I mentioned in the opening sentences of this chapter, what happens in reality, those contingencies that broad historicizing processes just cannot account for are perhaps even more revealing of the actual status quo of interventions. In the case of the rise and spread of CHWs within South Africa, one vignette will highlight the extreme level of precariousness or "thin citizenship" that CHWs (as an entire group and as a consequence of the AIDS industry) are exposed to.

Fluctuations of community health work

Lay health work or health volunteerism is not a new phenomenon in South Africa nor in the global context. In fact, it has a rather extensive history (De Wet, 2010; Van Ginneken et al., 2010) that has led to increasingly situating community health work within periodizations, thus historicizing this process by taking into account influential contextual forces that shaped its appearance over the years. On paper, it seems as if CHWs occupy an ever-developing and indispensable position in the national health force in South Africa to-day. A plethora of information now informs us of many facets of CHWs: their trajectories, roles, functions, outcomes, and challenges. Important issues, like that of CHW governance, are nascent and increasingly gaining attention (Schneider & Nxumalo, 2017; Schneider, 2019). In short supply are enquiries that deal with legitimizing CHWs' place within the healthcare environment (Mundeva et al., 2018), as well as deliberations to respond to the precariousness of their work situation and their struggle to gain legitimacy within existing trade union movements (Hlatshwayo, 2018). Given this state of nonrecognition, 2016 witnessed the launch of the National Union of Care Workers of South Africa (Trafford et al., 2018). The main focus of this newly formed union is to secure "decent work"[3] for this emerging health worker cadre.

Given their numbers and increasing importance granted to them (as will be discussed shortly), CHWs supposedly occupy a very important role in the South African healthcare landscape. Already in the early 2000s, a national framework emanating from the South African National Department of Health acknowledged the central position that CHWs occupy in the overall health system. Their deployment should also be seen in light of severe Human Resources for Health shortages in South Africa where in 2016, as reported in parliament, there was an estimated shortage of 44,780 nurses in the country (in Hlatshwayo, 2018). As early as 2004, a framework for CHW stipends (a form of remuneration) was produced. Despite the forewarning that CHWs should not be seen as a panacea to a dysfunctional healthcare system (Haines et al., 2007), the deployment of CHW is largely envisioned to bring about more equitable and efficient health services to the entire South African population as they are seen to be able to provide both preventive and curative functions.

The CHW program occupies a central position within the South African primary health care (PHC) reengineering approach that was announced by the former Minister of Health, Dr Aaron Motsoaledi, in 2011. The reengineering encompasses three "streams" of activities. First, it encompasses the creation of new ward-based PHC outreach teams and stipulates that there should be at least one of these PHC outreach teams per municipal ward (of which there are approximately 4,277; Malan, 2014b). The other two streams are focused on improving and expanding school health services and the creation of district-based specialist teams to curb the unacceptable high levels of child and maternal mortality in most of South Africa's districts[4] (Pillay & Barron, 2011).

The municipal ward-based primary health care outreach teams (WBPHCOTs) is an approach that is greatly inspired by the Brazilian model of outreach teams of health providers,[5] and in South Africa, the health ministry developed this novel PHC reengineering strategy in the context of broader reforms under the banner of Universal Health Coverage, better known as the "National Health Insurance" (Schneider et al., 2015). This document stipulates the core role that CHWs would play in these outreach teams (Department of Health, 2015). The deployment of the CHW program forms part of the broader vision toward more equitable healthcare within South Africa. This is because healthcare is still characterized by jarring disparities between those who can afford private medical care through contributing to medical aid schemes and those (the great majority of South Africans) reliant on the public healthcare system. According to Pillay and Barron (2011), the reengineering of the PHC is set to contribute to one of government's central strategies, namely "A Long and Healthy Life for All South Africans." An agreement (the negotiated service delivery agreement – NSDA) was consequently signed with the highest power in South Africa (the president), in which he committed himself as well as the Members of the Executive Council (MEC) of South Africa's nine provinces to attain four main outcomes, which are "to increase life expectancy; to decrease child and maternal mortality; to combat the HIV/AIDS epidemic and to lessen the burden of disease from TB; and lastly, to strengthen Health System Effectiveness" (Pillay & Barron, 2011).

This PHC reengineering specifically related to the creation of WBPHCOT is taking place in a context of already existing CHW activities. In fact, more than 72,000 community and facility-based lay workers connected to health departments were recorded by a government audit performed in 2011 (Schneider et al., 2015). These lay workers became active in health-related work in the wake of soaring HIV and tuberculosis (TB) prevalence in the early 2000s when there was little else to provide those with full-blown AIDS apart from palliative care and psychosocial support, and this care was mostly provided by these lay workers. In South Africa during this time, healthcare facilities were simply not capable of responding to the huge demand of care that HIV and its opportunistic infections brought about. Government officials started glorifying the work of lay healthcare workers through an array of rhetoric to persuade people to care for "their" ill community members (De Wet, 2010, 2011). This unwieldy and disease-specific domain of CHW that originated in post-apartheid South Africa is now increasingly harnessed and focused on to become a reorganized entity of uniform and standardized WBPHCOTs.

Each team will be responsible for a set number of households and will report to the local health facility. The roles ascribed to these outreach teams are comprehensive,

> Extending beyond HIV/TB to include maternal-child health and chronic non-communicable diseases; they will have a preventive and promotive orientation, and with other sectors and community based providers, will address social determinants of health.
>
> (National Department of Health, 2010,
> in Schneider et al., 2015)

Evidence abounds in gray literature, as well as in academic resources as to the positive results that emanate when using lay healthcare workers, widely known under the umbrella term of CHWs to contribute to the attainment of certain elusive public health goals that are often notoriously difficult to achieve (Perry & Zulliger, 2012). Instances of improved infant and maternal health outcomes linked to CHW activity in underserved areas have proven to be the most convincing evidence that this form of intervention has the potential to be effective (Lewin et al., 2012; Gilmore & McAuliffe, 2013). Choosing the route of community healthcare in settings where there are severe shortages is, therefore, ideal. Moreover, community mobilization, of which CHW programs are the zenith, was advocated by the UNAIDS and World Health Organization (WHO) as a "targeted strategic investment approach" toward combating HIV and AIDS (Schwartländer et al., 2011). The idea of using laypeople to provide healthcare dates back to the 1920s when in China, ordinary citizens were used to provide basic healthcare needs to the entire citizenry which culminated in the "barefoot doctor" or the "Cooperative Medical System" program that gained ascendency in the 1950s (Rifkin, 2008). It is purported that CHWs are instrumental to promote healthy behaviors among communities, on the one hand, and also to extend the reach of the healthcare system and, therefore, strengthening this important system, on the other (Perry et al., 2014). The simplicity of some interventions driven by these community health agents[6] is astounding. Modest interventions including correctly timed washing of hands, administering micronutrient supplements to children or oral rehydration therapy in cases of diarrhea, and psychosocial support to mostly underserved populations are but a few examples that have proven to save lives.

However, history tells a tale of complications and failures as to the implementation and seeming sustainability of CHW programs worldwide. An intervention deemed so simple and "normalized" has proven extremely arduous and unsuccessful to universally apply and sustain as can be witnessed by the waxing and waning of interests around CHW programs globally. It is argued that insufficient evidence records the overall effectiveness of CHW programs (Perry, 2013). However, it also seems that despite some proof of CHWs' efficiency in delivering positive health-related outcomes, the argument is continually made that there still seems to be an insufficient amount of information about their day-to-day activities and tasks as they are "poorly understood, not consistently documented, [and that there is] no harmonization as to [their] utilization, remuneration, retention" (Mwai et al., 2013).

Despite the fact that the concept of CHW is gaining increasing legitimacy in varied settings including their official recognition and role in US legislation,[7] the CHW context is by no means an uncontested and standard domain in the provision of healthcare. Numerous factors have been identified as constituting the root cause of difficulties associated with this cadre of healthcare worker. Ironically, its main weakness can probably be attributed to one of its greatest strengths: in its diversity and informality, CHWs probably often lose focus of their designated tasks. In contexts of numerous competing urgencies all clambering for attention, it is undoubtedly difficult to concentrate on one task only, as is often expected by the strict and bureaucratically aligned outlines of so-called job descriptions and the formalities of funding and government agencies and outcome-oriented results. When reading about the problems that plagued CHW programs in the 1980s, at a time when PHC soared to prominence after the much-vaunted and idealistic Alma Ata Declaration aiming for "Health for All by 2000," it is alarming to note how history seems to repeat itself. The problems faced in the 1980s are, to a large degree, identical to the problems these programs experience today and include,

> Inadequate training, insufficient remuneration or incentives for CHWs, and lack of supervision and logistical support for supplies and medicines. Programs were also plagued by deficient continuing education, poor integration with the health system, and lack of acceptance by higher-level healthcare providers. Additionally, in many programs, political favoritism led to inappropriate selection of CHWs.
>
> (Rifkin, 2008)

Another set of critique from a source conceived as long ago as 1989, could have been written about the state of CHWs today,

> CHW programs were conceived and developed as "vertical" programs, with little reference to existing health systems. Unlike other vertical programs, however, they had little extra funding. The programs were grafted onto, rather than integrated into, existing health systems. They were largely imposed from the center as a national response to an international emphasis on primary health care.
>
> (Gilson et al., 1989)

The foundering of the "health for all" vision in the 1970s was greatly ascribed to the lack of actual funding stipulations and commitments to implement this new vision for PHC and lay health worker utilization. This omission, combined with the 1980s debt crisis as well as a toned-down version of PHC called "selective primary health care" (Basilico et al., 2013), ushered in the failure of the Alma Ata PHC dream. Although intended as an "interim strategy" during a period of "diminished resources," the approach[8] of selective PHC attracted widespread support from mainly western (donor) nations as it provided clearer guidelines as to cost-effective health intervention packages that would yield "high returns in lives saved per dollar spent" (Basilico et al., 2013).

All of this points to the fact that interests and investments coupled with health-related tasks performed by laypeople are often congruent with wider global sentiments about the manner in which healthcare should be delivered. The vision for primary healthcare as envisioned in the 1970s was in line with extending care into communities to respond not only to healthcare needs but also to remedy generalized inequities in a variety of indicators, healthcare access being only one of the many skewed developmental outcomes among populations all over the world. This idealistic approach also echoes the preoccupation with addressing social determinants of health but was viewed with much suspicion in the Cold War period by Americans who saw elements of communism in this communitarian vision of healthcare (Packard, 2006).

It has been mentioned and is a well-known fact that the latest interest in CHW programs was engendered, to a large degree, by an emergency response to the fast-mounting HIV and AIDS epidemic that especially manifested in sub-Saharan Africa since the late 1990s. But it is equally apparent (even in community health work approaches in the USA) that "most CHW functions are intricately linked to the rest of the peripheral health system," largely distinguished by lacking resources despite assertions of organizations, such as the WHO and the Global Health Alliance that CHW programs need to be incorporated into the "overall strategic planning for human resources for health for that country and that they should be coherently located in the wider health system" (Bhutta et al., 2010).

It cannot be emphasized more that the AIDS epidemic put a heavy toll on the already overstretched human resources for health in many countries, notably in sub-Saharan Africa. As a remedy to this situation, it was soon declared that CHWs form an integral part in combatting HIV and AIDS and were widely considered to be a "cornerstone to the HIV response by international organizations and funding agencies" (Wringe et al., 2010). This disease and its far-reaching ramifications greatly challenged goals set by the Millennium Development Goals (MDGs), and the deployment of lay health workers, despite "limited evidence" of their successes at scale, somehow completed the equation to reach ambitious health targets. The coining of lay work in the concept of "task-shifting" also propelled a growing interest and investment in this new cadre of healthcare delivery.[9] The year 1994 also marked the commitment of international agencies and nongovernmental organizations (NGOs) who agreed and signed onto the Greater Involvement of People with AIDS (GIPA) initiative. Those involved in community lay care and task shifting were often infected and/or affected by HIV and AIDS. A campaign was also launched to train one million CHWs in Africa –

one for every 650 rural inhabitants (onemillionhealthworkers.org; Earth Institute, 2011). It is, however, rather perplexing that the ambitious UN-AIDS' 90-90-90 treatment targets have not explicitly focused on CHWs as players to attain these goals (Schneider et al., 2016).

Internationally, programs were crafted, implemented, and evaluated in order to reach consensus in the development industry as to so-called international best practices and evidence-based interventions to be used as measures to inform decision making and funding of community health interventions. As in the years of selective PHC, the language of pragmatism increasingly filtered into intervention decisions despite discourses pointing at more idealized notions of community care. The global frenzy to meet the demands for community care is evident in the increase in research about CHWs. Examples of articles reporting on the activities of community health work abound especially since 2011 (Schneider et al., 2016). In their scoping article on CHWs in low- and middle-income countries, the authors show that "there was a nearly sevenfold growth in annual number of publications over the period (2005–2014) from 23 in 2005 to 156 in 2014," and that "half of the publications came from the African region."

It is, therefore, evident that HIV and AIDS together with global health (Chapter 2) definitely introduced not only a renewed but also an unprecedented preoccupation in lay health work and an exceptional awareness in the potential of lay worker deployment dawned on aid organization across the globe. The manner in which lay workers are perceived, however, has greatly persisted in the many years that have marked the fluctuating interest in this group of emerging workers, as will be discussed in the next section.

Ideal types of CHW as "tactical citizenship"

The inherent tensions in the scope of practice, as well as the origins and intentions of CHWs, have been present for some time as can be witnessed by the formative work of some authors, such as David Werner (1977) who wrote an article titled "The Village Health Worker – Lackey or Liberator?" The dichotomy was drawn and conceptualized early on: should CHWs be mustered in the service of vertical disease programs strictly focused on beneficial and measurable health-related results largely to remedy failing healthcare systems (referring to so-called lackeys), or should they be "change agents" with a wide-ranging agenda and a strong activist inclination, addressing the social determinants of health ("liberators")? This Manichean divide entrenched the conceptualization of CHWs for the next couple of years. Berman and colleagues (1987), in their article "Community-based Health Workers: Head Start of False Start towards Health for All?" also point to the dualistic manner in which CHWs were imagined: either as global success stories or as complete failures. Perry and colleagues (2013) ask whether CHWs serve as the "lowest rung in the ladder of a service delivery team or as a community leader advancing social change?" Fiedler (2000)'s article's title equally provides two options with which to adjudicate one simple intervention provided by CHWs in Nepal: "The Nepal National Vitamin A Program: Prototype to Emulate or Donor Enclave?" The suspicion related to the contradictions of global funding is evident in the latter title.

Do CHWs carry more legitimacy if they meet a set of required criteria in order to become a CHW (for example, in South Africa, it is often said that they need to have at least a Matric qualification),[10] or if they have grown into community health work "organically"? Should they be motivated by the prospect of future employment and a potential livelihood, or should their intentions be altruistically motivated and selfless (Maes, 2015)? It is clear that CHWs, *more so than other "professions"*, are caught between two moral economies and could even be steeped in moral contradictions. Vin Kim Nguyen (2010) in his research on the proliferation of informal groups entwined in the AIDS industry indicates this predicament by stating that, on the one hand,

> organizing communities of people living with HIV [or in our case, involved with HIV and AIDS] was about solidarity and self-help; on the other, well-meaning efforts to support "empowerment" with much needed material support and confessional technologies of the self, fostered competition and undermined trust.
>
> (Nguyen, 2010)

One idealization of community health work punctuates notions of "Ubuntu"[11] and altruism; the other, cut-throat competition to survive in the AIDS industry – to secure funding, to protect one's patient territory, and to claim the most "legitimacy" to be able to render this service that could potentially be rendered by anyone, given the little expertise associated with lay health work.

In a more nuanced, evidence-based rendition of CHW activities and realities, Van Pletzen et al. (2013) set out to describe the bulk of CHW activities in three regions of South Africa and thereby to construct a useful typology, not mutually exclusive, of CHW program orientation in the contemporary South African context. The first and most common orientation was linked to the provision on "direct services" which entails,

> (…) psychosocial support and relieving poverty through providing access to resources; activities mostly take place in clients' homes, but also in community settings or formal health facilities.

The second part of the typology refers to a "developmental orientation" which involves

> (…) capacity-building in communities for instance by training or supervising groups or organizations to conduct health education programs or income generating projects; activities mostly take place in community settings like NPO premises, schools (…).

The last part of this typology includes an "activist orientation" that refers to the one side of the simplistic dichotomy related to CHWs that pitches these workers as "liberators" or "agents of change" who are au fait with the social determinants of health and actively combating these structural features by education and engagement,

> (...) mobilizing communities to become aware of and exercise their health rights; activities mostly take place in the community settings or formal health facilities.
>
> (Van Pletzen et al., 2013)

The authors also show that this last part of the typology that includes a level of activism is most likely to be present among CHWs who work at nonprofit organizations (NPOs) that are urban based and well to moderately resourced. In the rural and semi-rural areas, activism was practically nonexistent indicating that the dichotomy that started to take shape around CHW activities since the 1980s is largely irrelevant in the wider CHW context of the present.

Although the focus for CHWs in the Alma Ata Declaration was mainly on community involvement in prevention and promotion, this focus shifted rather dramatically with the challenges that started mounting to attain the outcomes of the health MDGs and the recent shift in sub-Saharan countries toward using CHWs to increase access to ART (Bennet et al., 2014). Moreover, the interplay and tensions between these two idealized notions seem to become increasingly problematic as disease burdens just get heavier in resource-constrained settings,

> As low- and middle-income countries confront a new generation of health challenges such as non-communicable diseases, mental health and violence and injury, the repertoire of possible CHW roles is ever-expanding. There is a danger of role fragmentation and overload and a need to re-think roles in new and more complex ways. (...) Similarly, strategies of specialization and the balance between disease-specific and integrated approaches need to be defined. In the process, there is the risk that the social and environmental health roles of CHWs get crowded out by technical and treatment roles of core cadres, especially if the latter are incentivized.
>
> (Schneider et al., 2016)

Adding complexity to the conceptualization of CHW also emerged by those who have identified "hidden" layers of community-based health delivery (Leon et al., 2015). In the process of adhering to conceptualized dichotomies, we can lose sight of other cadres of workers who also make a potential contribution to serving marginalized communities but who are not necessarily "counted" in as much as they are not trained, administered, remunerated, or monitored.

As with ART providing a good chance of survival to those with HIV, participation in and association with HIV organizations also allows unprecedented opportunities to access some of the potential material benefits and opportunities that could be lifesaving in contexts of severe precarity. Stipends, new networks of support, prospects of training and job security, and amassing valuable experience are all bread-and-butter issues that CHWs are faced with on an everyday basis. By becoming CHWs, these individuals are potentially also exercising "tactical citizenship" (Nguyen, 2010) where there is a blurring of egoistic and altruistic motives to become *and to remain* a CHW. A critique of the dichotomous manner that greatly portrays and thereby confines thinking about CHWs was also developed in a more recent article by Colvin and Swartz (2015), the title also reflecting what has become according to the authors, a "reified" dichotomy, "Community Extension Agents or Agents of Change? Community Health Workers and the Politics of Care Work in Postapartheid South Africa." The authors depict the limitations of this narrow bifurcated approach by critiquing the fact that such a rigid understanding of their role does not take into account CHWs' real experiences and contemporary contexts that greatly shape the manner in which these practices continue to evolve.

Max Weber too rejected the view that human phenomena are always and exclusively "historical" inasmuch as phenomena obtain their significance "only from the precise where, when and how of their once-off occurrence" (Harrington, 2005). This famous theorist was of the opinion that all scientific discourse aims to use generally accepted concepts to ensure a level of continuity of individual cases with more generally recurrent phenomena. There were, however, two significant criterions that marked what Weber called "the science of culture." First, those concepts employed in the "sciences of culture" have no intention to devise "general laws of human conduct, much less of laws of historical development" (Harrington, 2005). Second, the concepts that characterize the "sciences of culture" are not comparable to the concepts utilized in the natural sciences. Weber emphasized that concepts used in the "sciences of culture" are *ideal-typical concepts.* These ideal types constitute "possible confluences of concepts or typologies, which can be used by the scholar to analyze and categorize particular features of the subject matter under consideration" (Harrington, 2005). Ideal types should, therefore, be seen to act merely as tools of analysis inasmuch as "they do not express a judgement about what is 'ideal' in a phenomenon in the sense of intrinsically worthy or admirable." I would suggest then that these ideal types that have been created through the conceptualization of CHWs should be expanded and should take into account the contingencies that come to shape the lived realities of CHWs in South Africa and beyond, thereby juxtaposing the ideal-typical with that of the real.

The critique against this dichotomous reading which greatly effaces the real-life experiences of CHWs is in line with Nguyen (2010), resonating with the introductory reference to Achille Mbembe's emphasis, that *contingency* plays as much a role in the development of "glocal"[12] interventions of community health work. Nguyen states that "voluntary associations [many of which are active in the domain of health care] were [and still are] in some ways social laboratories, allowing new forms of social organization to be experimented with and to spread" (Nguyen, 2010).

Therefore, the origin and development of CHWs as we have come to know them today is largely as a result of historical but also complex and unique circumstantial and accidental events as well as responses to these events. People, especially when faced with extreme forms of precarity, embrace opportunities to become active as volunteers or CHWs in the context of HIV and AIDS for an array of understandable reasons. These reasons span the continuum from mere opportunism to selfless altruism. But also, the proliferation of volunteer organizations where those most affected with HIV and AIDS could be reached and organized was largely based on experience and examples from the global North (especially America and Europe), where it was demonstrated that this kind of association had the potential to lead to stronger solidarity and a "sense of community" between those who are infected, as well as affected with HIV and AIDS (Nguyen, 2010). However, for these volunteers who eventually became known as CHWs, strict requirements had to be adhered to in order to be recognized and to be recipients even of meager and erratic assistance (mostly financial, the infamous "stipends"). CHWs, especially those who were living with HIV, had to "disclose" and deliver testimonials in order to proof that this would lead to "positive living." Nguyen (2010) shows how these requirements were often devised in contexts far away from the realities of those infected and affected with HIV and AIDS in Africa, but that this had somehow become the gold standard of best practices in these mushrooming associations that were predominantly vying for financial assistance. Nguyen's (2010) ethnography craftily shows the manner in which voluntary associations often became "mechanisms for palliating economic insecurity; [...] ultimately they were spaces where a form of politics could be fashioned." This brief outline of the contexts, expectations, conceptualizations, and contradictions creates the backdrop against which the trajectory of contemporary CHWs in South Africa should be viewed.

In the previous section, we witnessed the shortfalls that accompany the conceptualization of CHW in a simplistic, binary manner. Becoming a CHW, and somehow sculpting the way in which they go about their work and develop their own "professional" identity is an example of "self-fashioning" as purported by Achille Mbembe (2002). The increase in CHW organizations – voluntary in many instances, but remunerated at times albeit sporadically and erratically – pried open an opportunity for new forms of "tactical citizenship," where unemployed and destitute women (most CHW are female) could start participating in an "informal" or "parallel" economy as a novel way to assuring a more secure form of citizenship. Them opting and acting as CHWs, and making strategic decisions in their day-to-day lives, indicates their own agency in *being* CHWs, and somehow exacting new forms of participation in "the existential achievements of public participation" in this "newfound pleasures of civic virtue" (Steinberg, 2016). South Africa experiences widespread and bothersome unemployment. With a rate of over 27% unemployment, any opportunity to perform a "job" is understandably an opportune occurrence (Fin24, 2019). The advent of the new wave of interest and investment in community health work took root in this context of dire need. This need primarily manifests at the level of income. Any source of income is timely, even if not always reliable. Even the prospect of income is better than nothing at all. However, employment offers more than just remuneration. It could lead to a sense of belonging, to feelings of worth, and to other positive mind-sets. Job insecurity has been associated with a perceived loss of a person's social identity (Selenko et al., 2017). It has been shown that volunteers' (or CHWs')

> personal identity and values (views of self as an individual), and role identity as a volunteer and the group identity of the organization were linked. The consistency between organizational values and member values is an important factor in increasing individuals' identification with the organization.
>
> (Naidu et al., 2012)

However, as Achille Mbembe indicates, among current conditions from which Africans fashion their identities, there is a prevalent condition that he calls "the state of war." Mbembe (2002) argues that "the state of war" in contemporary Africa should, in fact, be conceived of as a "general cultural experience that shapes identities, just as the family, the school, and other social institutions do" (in Tembo, 2018). There is cruelty and lawlessness that characterize this "state of war." This state is "a zone of indistinction" where "decisions about life and death become entirely arbitrary" (Mbembe, 2002). The conditions of current CHWs in South Africa, together with a vignette that will follow thereafter, emphasize this "state of war" under which CHWs fashion their selves – an example of exercising a form of citizenship in conditions of precarity, or in other words, a quintessential manifestation of "thin citizenship."

CHWs in post-apartheid South Africa

As indicated before, our country's own CHW trajectory is rather unique, given that it started at a time of the South African government's denialist stance toward HIV etiology and the associated unwillingness to avail ART to those in need of them. The first CHWs were thus focused on providing, what was euphemistically called "palliative" home-based care, on the one hand, and to expand and perform DOTS interventions for those afflicted by TB, on the other (Schneider et al., 2016). Only with the much-awaited arrival of ART did their "roles shift towards home-based HIV-testing; referral for, or home initiation of ART; and community-based adherence support and follow-up of care for ART and TB treatment, increasingly as integrated programs" (Schneider et al., 2016). This cursory view of the emergence of CHWs in South Africa since the end of apartheid is indicative of the fact that any CHW program is extremely context specific (Kok et al., 2015), which makes any attempt at standardized approaches (the dominant way in which to go about developing interventions) very complicated and prone to failure. The international stars of evidence-based improvements in multi-faceted health outcomes provided by lay health workers are widely cited in the dominant literature. Countries such as Ethiopia, Mali, Niger, and India (Leon et al., 2015) with much lower per capita spending on health compared to South Africa are seeing substantially more positive outcomes compared to a relatively affluent country like South Africa. This is noteworthy given the South African state's actions to create a large cadre of standardized CHWs as an essential component of the WBPHCOT initiative under the PHC reengineering process that is slowly and tentatively emerging in South Africa.

It is a truism, often reiterated in academic discourses, that a sound relationship between CHWs and the overall health system is paramount when it comes to the solidification of CHW legitimacy in the eyes of the wider community as well as forging their own perceptions of their roles and responsibilities (Perry et al., 2013). Perry et al. (2013) have indicated that within stronger health systems, it is more likely that CHW programs are "indistinguishable from the rest of the system." In cases where the health systems are fragile and resources are limited, "CHW programs are often created as add-ons intended to increase coverage or address unmet health needs and are inadequately integrated with the broader health system" (Perry et al., 2013). A flaw in the system that dictates CHW activities, roles, responsibilities, and accountability, but also their worth and value, has the far-reaching potential to de-legitimize CHWs to a great extent. The heterogeneous CHW sorority has an uphill battle in this quest for legitimacy as the health system in South Africa is notoriously hierarchical and where there is widespread lack of respect from professional health staff cadres because of CHWs' lower status, prevalent gender bias, their precarious socioeconomic status, and the marked educational differences between CHWs and other healthcare professionals (Perry et al., 2013).

Despite these challenges, this informal cadre of work increased tremendously since the early 2000s and started occupying an ever-expanding position within the imaginary and real spaces of the healthcare system. On paper at least, as early as 2012, the Department of Health's *Human Resources for Health* report indicated that planning around CHWs would include "develop[ing] the training infrastructure, plans, reimbursements and career pathways for CHWs" (in Trafford et al., 2018). At first, funding for the CHW programs was secured through a variety of sources including the Expanded Public Works Program (EPWP) as well as "national ring fenced grants for HIV and TB" which provided the necessary basis from which this service platform could continue and expand. In current times of increased access to treatment and generalized normalization, "the focus of home based shifted to de-hospitalized care of other chronic diseases, adherence support for those on ART and TB treatment, and most recently, school health services" (Schneider et al., 2015). However, it has been found that costs associated with the operation of effective CHW program are frequently much greater than initially anticipated (Perry et al., 2013). There was the welcome announcement during the 2019 Budget Speech by the current minister of Finances, Tito Mboweni, that an additional R1 billion was earmarked to increase the wages of CHWs to the level of the basic minimum wage which amounts to R3,500 per month (South African Government News Agency, 2019).

With the ambitious vision of the South African Department of Health to achieve universal healthcare, CHWs are seen – perhaps more than ever – to occupy a central role in imagining the reformulation of policies and the development of primary healthcare. Universal healthcare, as championed by the Department of Health, is aspired to by securing increased state health financing through an ambitious National Health Insurance scheme and by developing the reengineering of PHC. This reengineering, as was discussed earlier on, will then render CHWs central to the new ward-based outreach teams that will be serving groups within communities.[13] But according to Trafford et al. (2018), this new strategy that implicates CHWs leads to even further complications within an "uneven and fragmented landscape of CHW roles, employment conditions, and relationships with other health system role players." The development of the much-vaunted PHC reengineering policy has been slow, consultations inconsistent and insufficient, and dissemination poor (Trafford et al., 2018). Implementation plans have not been produced despite the fact that the PHC reengineering has kicked off at various sites. Practically speaking, though, studies have found that within South Africa,

> (…) their roles, particularly in households, were often vague and lacking in definition, tending to follow a limited number of locally mandated routines, and heavily focused on meeting daily visit quotas. Patient journeys and observations documented large numbers of missed opportunities for intervention (in all age groups) within households. A significant part of the day, especially in rural areas, was consumed with walking to and from the homes of the patients.
>
> (Schneider et al., 2015)

Perhaps the most troubling absence in the extensive range of knowledge related to CHW and their activities is the fact that little evidence is available to direct and forewarn as to the management of CHW programs *at scale*, something that the national South African government is currently in the process of developing (Schneider et al., 2015). Equally worrying in the case of South Africa's move toward a universal CHW program are the associated challenges of reorientating a range of eclectic community-based services that literally sprung up overnight to respond to disease-specific requirements notably related to HIV and AIDS and to TB and to the creation of a standardized and regulated CHW program.

There are plenty of hazards in the processes that would mark the implementation of the new policy guidelines to reengineer PHC in South Africa. One important risk identified by Schneider et al. (2015) is that funding could be reoriented from supporting informal NPOs and thereby using these funds to strengthen state-run national health programs (this did happened post-1994). This will be a deathblow to independent NPOs, as these organizations will then automatically be without required resources or experienced staff. In many instances, NPOs currently fulfill tasks that will not necessarily be covered by the newly formed ward-based outreach teams, which will be detrimental to communities who benefit from these services and networking in the NPO sector. Moreover, those community-based organizations with a critical inclination, if amalgamated within the state's reengineering plans, will find it increasingly difficult to act as "watchdogs" in a climate of dependency (Schneider et al., 2015). The general "lay of the land" of contemporary CHW realities was sketched in this section, which further entrenches the levels of "thin citizenship" that characterizes those associated with the AIDS industry in contemporary South Africa.

The story of the Free State province's CHW program

On 16 April 2014, the former Free State Health Department MEC (Member of the Executive Council), Benny Malakoane, issued an abrupt circular that, in effect, fired 3,800 lay workers. The memo was sent to "Directors of Programs, District Managers, CEO's, Program Managers and Community Liaison Officers." The subject of the memo was longer than the content thereof, stating that it consists of "Services offered by community volunteers paid by HIV & AIDS Grant and EPWP; Home-based Carers and their Supervisors; DOTS Supporters; Medical Male Circumcision field workers; High Transmission Area field workers; Lay Counsellors; Peer Educators and Support Group Facilitators" (this in itself indicating the complexity of the tasks and denominations that accompany this cadre of lay workers).

The content of the memo first deals with the finalization of outstanding stipend payments for the months of March and April 2014, which is stated, would be paid by the end of April 2014. It then proceeds to state that notice should be taken that "all volunteers should stop their services by 30 April 2014." It then continues with an incomplete elucidation "the Department will embark on the new system of partnering with NGOs and working with the volunteers." It bizarrely ends by stating: "Note that this excludes the Community Health Workers."

Although not mentioned in this memo, it later came to light that this drastic action was also made possible and justified because of "new criteria" in formalizing this cadre of lay health workers – one of which stipulates CHWs' ages, specifying that most of the CHWs who were fired were actually "too old" and were deemed as having an "under-educated status" notwithstanding the fact that some of these CHWs had been fulfilling this function for several years (Cullinan & Nkosi, 2015). The Free State province in South Africa unfortunately has a terrible track record when it comes to health outcomes and performance.[14] Although it is the second smallest province by population, the province has historically featured poorer health outcomes compared to the rest of South Africa and, as far back as 1996, has consistently been ranked with the lowest life expectancy at birth. The province has 31 public healthcare facilities that provide services to the great majority of the province's population. In 2008, a crisis in funding caused major problems with the supply of drugs to the extent that a moratorium had to be placed on the procurement of ART. This moratorium lasted four months and resulted in an estimated 30 deaths per day (Spotlight, 2016). In February 2015, doctors working in public healthcare facilities all over the province made public their grievances by providing incriminatory evidence of the dire state of this healthcare sector (Van Wyk & Brodie, 2015). It was found that in 2015, the total number of doctors working in the public healthcare sector in the Free State dropped to 539 from 716 in 2014. This 24% reduction happened at a time when the province had a ratio of only 23.3 doctors per 100,000 patients. In 2016, the Free State Department of Health was placed under administration, with National Treasury taking responsibility for its budget.

It is within this broader context of sub-standard healthcare provision, allegations of corruption, stock-outs, and patient complaints that the issue of the categorical suspension of lay workers has to be understood. Their suspension led to a delegation of CHWs together with the activist group, the Treatment Action Campaign (TAC), to request a meeting with the provincial MEC for Health and signatory of the memo that dismissed them. The TAC wrote in a statement that the workers

> were protesting [against] the state of the public healthcare system in the Free State, their conditions of employment and the decision of the MEC for the Free State department of health, Benny Malakoane, to effectively terminate their employment without warning.
>
> (Green, 2015)

The attempt to organize a meeting with the MEC was, however, not successful and culminated into a decision to stage a series of protests of CHWs together with the TAC. A peaceful vigil to the provincial department of health's headquarters in Bloemfontein, Bophelo House, resulted in the arrest of 127 of these CHWs in June 2014. These arrested CHWs were charged with the dated, apartheid-era crime of participating in an illegal activity. To be more specific, they were accused of contravening the Regulations of Gatherings Act 205 of 1993. Some of those arrested were elderly women who, after their arrest, had to spend 36 hours in cells, while many were detained without access to their chronic medicines.

The case was postponed seven times after the initial written submission to the National Director of Public Prosecutions to drop the charges against the group of CHWs. The logistics involved to get all 94 accused to convene in Bloemfontein from all corners of the province's 129,825 km^2 cost the defense a great amount of money and logistical organization. Another reason for the frequent postponement of the case was the fact that there were 94 CHWs who stood accused of this offense, while some of the CHWs (approximately 30) agreed to a settlement with the state (to plead guilty to the charges).[15] The magistrate's court facilities also could not cater for the logistical needs of such a high number of accused to appear in court all at once. One magistrate postponed the trial after indicating that "this is not a humane or dignified manner to conduct a trial. I see people struggling to breathe and fanning themselves" (Health E-News, 2015). In fact, the court case was postponed several times, only starting on their sixth appearance and continuing to a seventh. The case dragged on for two long weeks. Section 27 expressed their outrage at the testimony from the Public Order Police over those five days. It so transpired that this police unit

> repeatedly explained how they routinely – as per a long-held institutional practice – make unlawful arrests, violate the rights to freedom of expression and demonstration, and use apartheid-era means of crowd control. In the course of their testimony, it became obvious that this case is about more than a disagreement between a few gogos[16] and an MEC – it is about a serious threat to a right fundamental to a free society.
>
> (Section 27, 2015)

It transpired in the court proceedings that the healthcare workers believed that they were being punished not for breaking some or other law but for having publicly dared to defy the MEC of Health (and thereby, government). In fact, they were exercising a form of activism (or active citizenship) by speaking out. Their quest was rooted in their preoccupation with the conditions of healthcare not only for their "patients," on the one hand, but also for the possibility to continue with their "jobs," their lifeline, and their sense of identity and belonging, on the other.

The civil organization group, Section 27, strongly condemned this action by the state:

> The state's disproportionate response to a group of mainly aged women peacefully singing and praying at a night vigil remains hard to explain – especially since it is now clear that even the police did not consider there to be any actual threat to public safety or to property. The state's decision then to prosecute and to spend what must be hundreds of thousands of Rands on the prosecution is even more irrational, especially in light of the scarcity of public resources.
>
> (Section 27, 2015)

Despite this argument and the contrived manner in which the prosecution utilized this dated legislation, on 1 October 2015, all 94 of the accused CHWs (the so-called Bophelo House 94) were found guilty in the Bloemfontein Magistrate's Court of attending a gathering for which no notice was given. The defense also argued that the vigil posed no threat to public safety or to property. The judge in the trial, Magistrate Thafeni, ruled that this specific gathering was "prohibited" as no notice was provided to the police (Section 27, 2015). On 2 October 2015, she sentenced the Bophelo House 94 to a fine of R600 or three months imprisonment, both suspended for three years provided that they do not violate Section 12(1)(e) of the Gatherings Act. This judgment, by implication, would mean that any meeting of more than 15 people without prior notification to the police could be considered a "prohibited" gathering and would, therefore, be unlawful. John Stephens of Section 27 indicated that

> the judgement amounts to a requirement, in essence, that people can only exercise their rights when given express permission to do so, a particularly frightening requirement in the context of the right to protest. This understanding of the law is eerily akin to apartheid's infamous Internal Security Act and is diametrically opposed to the current state of the law under the Regulation of Gatherings Act. The police seem to be applying the law in this way across the province [Free State province]. Just recently, approximately 30 health activists in Reitz were arrested for similar reasons. It is abundantly clear that these arrests intend to stifle dissent and assembly, the precise rights the Gatherings Act is meant to manage and protect.
>
> (Stephens, 2015)

In a similar vein, the words of Anele Yawa, the General Secretary of the TAC, echo the disbelief in such a practice of the law as "it makes a mockery of our constitutionally guaranteed right to peaceful protest. It is a judgement that you would expect in a police state, not a constitutional democracy" (Section 27, 2015). This is especially so given the mechanistic reading by the judge of this Act, for it was indisputably demonstrated that no special circumstances characterized this gathering, none that could warrant the definition thereof in terms of needing to have been prohibited. This shocking judgment encouraged the lawyers of the Bophelo House 94 to appeal the judgment in the High Court. In the words of the TAC's Anele Yawa,

> This prosecution is not about justice. Instead, this case is about punishing those who dare speak out – and challenge power – about their unfair dismissal and the dysfunction in the Free State public healthcare system. The arrests and the prosecution is a flagrant abuse of the state apparatus and aims to suppress healthy democratic dissent. We will appeal this judgment in the interests of all people in South Africa in order to make clear that the right to assemble cannot be violated in this way. An injury to one is an injury to all.
>
> (Section 27, 2015)

The political undercurrents of this event were clearly visible. Section 27 and the TAC made no secret of their suspicion of the workings within the Free State Department of Health.[17] In a December 2016 article, they explicitly stated that since 2008, there was a positive and cooperative relationship with the then national Minister of Health, Dr Aaron Motsoaledi, and his predecessor, Barbara Hogan. According to these activist groups, both these ministers are "visionary and committed." They did, however, state that it was clear that these ministers' "hands are tied" when it comes to effectuating important decision making and action, and that "provinces are able to call the shots" (Thom & Heywood, 2016). Among health activists and doctors, it is said that Malakoane (the former provincial health MEC) and the Free State province's former Premier, Ace Magashule, are "higher up in the ANC ranks than Motsoaledi," and that this is largely the reason why some actions cannot be condemned publically (Malan, 2015). The TAC published scathing accounts of the former health MEC and other highly placed officials, reporting on a series of issues that tarnished the reputation of these officials (TAC & Section 27, 2016a).[18] The TAC, together with the assistance of pro bono legal representation, took the matter on appeal in August 2016.

In November 2016, more than two years after the arrest of the CHWs, a "landmark judgement" set aside the convictions and sentences of the 94 accused. This ruling was an important precedent to protect people's right to protest as it was found that the "draconian" apartheid-era legislation that the CHWs were charged with of contravening was archaic in South Africa's post-apartheid context and the rights that all South Africans now equally enjoy under the banner of our progressive Constitution. However, it was a dear price to pay by CHWs, some who lost their sole potential of attaining some form of "employment" and the accompanying material and psychological benefits of their former positions.[19] It was stated in the joint statement by the TAC and Section 27 that the ruling confirmed their view that all along, the prosecution of the CHWs was a politically motivated action and that state resources were abused in the protracted process of court cases being postponed and all the other shenanigans that characterized the case since 2014 (TAC & Section 27, 2016b).

This vignette powerfully depicts the "thin citizenship" and precarity that are at play in the vicissitudes and the contingencies within programs that were borne from the exceptional AIDS era, in this case, the proliferation of the CHW program across South Africa. This is but one vignette, an example of events that are certainly more widespread in contexts of high disease burdens and constrained resources. This vignette could be described and told simply because of its media visibility and the fact that activist groups could muster the resources to speak truth to power. Many of these stories are unfortunately never told. It is a strong reminder of the manner in which Africans (in a time of AIDS but also now in a time of HIV), in a quest of self-actualization and applying strategic agency to enhance forms of citizenship and belonging, are mostly doing so in conditions of the "state of war" (Mbembe's analogy described earlier). It has also been demonstrated that a phenomenon as complex as the proliferation of lay healthcare workers (the variations of which are hard to capture and standardize) is forced into static and simplistic definitions and tasks that respond to the dictates – currently the gold standard of interventions – of evidence-based results and cost-effectiveness. These rational and calculated formulations of complex activities open opportunities to use and abuse people *legitimately*. Perhaps, I entertain a too mechanistic and rational reading of the happenings of the #BopheloHouse94, but I would suggest a reading of "collateral damage" of the events that led to the dismissal of the CHWs in 2014: The reengineering ward-based outreach team (WBOT) program allowed authorities in the Free State province an opportunity to dismiss these lay workers in the first place (as new requirements were stipulated in the recruitment of CHWs in the WBOT teams), although these reasons for the dismissal of the 129 CHWs were never explicitly stated. In fact, the process of standardization and implementation of CHW programs will lead to more unintended consequences and widespread anxiety among many people who were once made to believe that they were indispensable in the fight against AIDS (as explained earlier).[20] This inevitable rationalization and triage are both symptomatic of the wider context in which global health dictates reign supreme and where technological and "tame" interventions are privileged. Locally, as Jonny Steinberg (2016) has reasoned,

> AIDS medicine has become one of the many instruments through which the ANC government exerts soft power over the lives of the rural poor, binding them into a national project of expectation.

Not only the availability of AIDS medicines but also the associated activities, such as the possibility to work as a CHW in a WBPHCOT are characterized by the precariousness of bureaucratic processes linked to standardization, cost-effectiveness and policy dictates, often determined in places far removed from the local contexts in where these interventions are most needed.

The domino effect of events that led to the 2016 court ruling was symptomatic of local consequences of these global dictates, thereby adding another layer of complexity in making sense of the messy assemblages that the HIV and AIDS industry has given rise to.

Conclusion

Hypothetically, the use of CHWs is a response to foster more inclusive, participatory, equitable, and relevant reactions to healthcare needs in a world where inequalities are soaring unabatedly. From its early days, especially in the 1980s, a certain conceptualization started creating a tension between two ideal typical roles that CHWs could fulfill: mere "extra pairs of hands" ("lackeys"), on the one hand, or agents of change and activism ("liberators"), on the other. Unfortunately, the history of community-based healthcare activities is replete with the duplication of errors and falls prey to the pitfalls of the past.

CHWs have largely become part and parcel of the discourses and practices of rendering healthcare as is evident in the burgeoning literature that deals with their evaluation and analysis but also within policy documents and strategic future decision-making evident in South Africa through the development of the reengineered PHC approach. Some CHWs in South Africa, mostly women, have been actively doing CHW work for more than a decade now.[21] Many CHWs are seropositive but not all of them. However, what makes the rise of global health concomitant with the HIV epidemic so exceptional is the manner in which it simultaneously triaged those who were deemed deserving of care and treatment, on the one hand, and, on the other, opened up new opportunities not only for those infected but also those affected, to create new spaces of belonging and to develop to various degrees, claims to the precarious spoils of beneficence and philanthropy that the disease engendered.

But this "opening up of opportunities" comes with unexpected twists and turns. The capricious handling of CHWs as described in the earlier vignette juxtaposes the initial emergence of current CHW deployment – originally an offshoot of larger global and local shifts in harnessing informal healthcare. What happened to these arrested CHWs is indicative of the consequences, and not just of the fads of the AIDS industry, stretching much further to somehow highlight notions of self-fashioning in light of generalized precarity and the interplay between "strategic" and "thin" citizenship. Nguyen's view on this interplay (albeit with his focus on HIV-positive self-help groups and not CHW groups) is expressed in the following excerpt:

> The notion of citizenship highlights the political dimensions of the patterns of resort that brought people diagnosed with HIV to self-help groups and the social relations that resulted. These trajectories were attempts to influence fate, to enroll others in one's destiny, and to shape how the future played out in the organization of communities around HIV.
>
> (Nguyen, 2010)

The constant battle between these two forms of citizenship characterizes not only aspects of treatment access and physical survival but also wider initiatives that are obdurately part of the wider AIDS industry and that could be determining to "resist political and economic death and social oblivion" (Biehl & Petryna, 2013). In self-fashioning contexts defined by "contexts of war," the violence is always linked to the limited resources that are available. Often these resources that are available become subject to a calculus of need, interventions could also be stopped at any point in time, and newly fashioned livelihoods could face brusque elimination. CHWs are but one group entrapped in the vicissitudes of the AIDS industry because although they could be uninfected and physically well, they are more than often "economically dead" (Biehl, 2007). The fate of CHWs – infected or affected – if reliant on donor help or arbitrary (although seemingly "rational") government investment, is as much an exercise in deciding on issues of life and death and triage, as on procuring lifesaving treatment.

Notes

1   The concept of "thin citizenship" is developed by Vinh-Kim Nguyen (2010) to mark the vicissitudes of the struggle over "life itself" in a time of AIDS: rationed treatment, triage, and the exceptional exercise of sovereignty. Not only suffering from AIDS but also the manifold "AIDS derivatives" (Hunt, 1997) and its erratic nature (marked by abundance and scarcity), accentuate and bring to the fore more starkly, this notion of "thin citizenship."

2   The history of challenges associated with the correct place (hospitals or clinics?), and professionals (doctors, nurses, or CHWs?), to administer and to monitor treatment, is also indicative of a complex evolution of the manner in which HIV and AIDS was responded to and perceived by academics and the medical profession itself.

3   According to the International Labor Organization's website, "decent work" is defined as a situation that "involves opportunities for work that is productive and delivers a fair income, security in the workplace and social protection for families, better prospects for personal development and social integration, freedom for people to express their concerns, organize and participate in the decisions that affect their lives and equality of opportunity and treatment for all women and men" (International Labor Organization, n.d.).

4   This chapter will not discuss the other two streams of the PHC reengineering approach as the focus is specifically on CHW programs.

5   The one big difference with the Brazilian model is the fact that the South African ward-based teams do not include a medical doctor. The South African ward-based teams are composed of six CHWs who work under the surveillance of a professional nurse, accompanied by a health promotion and environmental officer (Malan, 2014b).

6   The appellation, *Agentes Comunitàrios de Saude*, or "community health agents," represents lay health workers active in one of the most prominent and successful CHW programs globally. Active in Brazil since the mid-1980s, this program comprises health teams that include professional healthcare practitioners and lay healthcare workers to reach the entire Brazilian population by doing home visits and rendering other services to 110 million people (Mayberry & Baker, 2011). In Brazil, an estimated 240,000 CHWs are active in this service that has seen marked improvements in population health status (Perry et al., 2014).

7   In the USA, known for its unequal healthcare system and inequities related to access to healthcare, CHWs were recognized in the Patient Protection and Affordable Care Act, passed as part of "Obamacare," to provide necessary health services to poor and underserved citizens and to lead to improvements in access to health and health outcomes of this segment of the population (Rosenthal et al., 2010). However, it is clear that this type of CHW program is not truly comparable to those that are often depicted under the banner of CHWs working in low- and middle-income countries.

8   One influential article by Julia Walsh and Kenneth Warren greatly set the scene for the adoption of progressive PHC (Walsh & Warren, 1979).

9   The term "task-shifting" was very fashionable after it popularization by organizations such as the WHO in their 2006 World Health Report which encouraged "community participation and systemic delegation of tasks to less specialized cadres." The WHO (2008) identified 313 tasks as "essential for the prevention of

HIV transmission, identification of HIV-positive individuals, provision of basic HIV clinical management, and initiation and maintenance of patients on ART." It is subsequently recommended that 115 of these tasks can be executed by CHWs (WHO, 2008). However, Lehman et al. (2009) are of the opinion that the process of implementing task-shifting and of involving a wide range of stakeholders did not happen. They indicate that task-shifting will thus "exist on the political and organizational periphery of the formal health system, exposed to policy and funding fashions, and become fragile and unsustainable."

10 "Matric" is the equivalent of the final year of secondary schooling. Grade 1 – Matric (or Grade 12) implies at least 12 years of schooling.

11 "Ubuntu" is a Nguni term which means "humanity" and is rooted in a philosophy of sharing that connects all humanity.

12 "Glocal" refers to the concept developed by Roland Robertson (1992) who explains globalization as a cultural process whereby there is an interpenetration of the global and local to potentially give rise to new forms of local culture or to bring about distinctive new combinations of this interactions (Robertson, 1992). Mbembe (2002) argues that "global practices of symbolic exchange have affected African lives in different spheres, including individual African identity. The result is a complex matrix from which Africans fashion their identities, and the intersection of global flows and local practices is the site of African identity formation."

13 Reports as to failures of the pilot WBPHCOT system roll-out have been reported: in the North West, it is estimated that the province lost more than 30 ward-based CHW teams and were forced to cut health posts in the province. The WBPHCOT pilot project in the Free State's Thabo Mofutsanyana district was also mired in failure.

14 A series of public hearings were organized by the TAC to collect ordinary citizens' stories related to deficient healthcare, drug stock-outs, and inhumane treatment in public healthcare facilities in the province. This damning document can be found online (TAC, 2018).

15 Initially, 129 CHWs stood accused of the contravention of Act 205 of 1993. According to a joint TAC/Section 27 statement, government forced some to sign statements to admit guilt for charges to be dropped. Some CHWs did agree to accept this plea bargain and, therefore, did not have to stand trial and potentially be sentenced. However, they now have a criminal record for this "contravention."

16 Meaning "old ladies" or "grandmas."

17 Their opposition to the former MEC of Health in the Free State province was rooted in the fact that he was also facing corruption charges although the charges had recently (in 2018) been dropped because of a lack of evidence against him.

18 It should be noted that these actions against the CHWs and the dire position of the Free State health system happen under the banner of ANC control, as this is the dominant party in the country and in the province. However, this party is also the party that provides the promises of "post-revolutionary upward mobility" (Steinberg, 2016).The promise of treatment and the promise of opportunities are firmly vested in the current status quo. Steinberg (2016) explicates the curious contradiction as developed by Albert Hirschman where he indicates that post-revolutionary societies often show inexplicable levels of tolerance to growing inequalities. This is partly to be explained by those "left behind" feeling bonded to the nouveaux riches and can thus "take an imagined journey on their coat-tails" (Steinberg, 2016). Also, Steinberg explains this in terms of older generations' powerful desire to witness generational improvement, even if it leads to increased inequality.

19 Some but not all of these CHWs were reinstated in their positions. The exact fate of each CHW is not known.

20 This interplay between the local and the global in terms of consequences is reminiscent of Zygmunt Bauman's (1998) analysis of the "human consequences of globalization."

21 Some authors are placing increasing emphasis on the fact that what was normally seen as the "feminization of poverty" has now also turned into the "feminization of responsibility" or "coerced agency" where it is often expected of women (and believed by women) that they have to take care of the family as well as the community. This is indicative of dominant notions of motherhood and religion which are strongly associated "characteristics" of women that often lie at the root of their decisions to volunteer. It is also indicated in some studies that men are often deterred from caring roles as these roles are too often perceived as belonging to the domain of women and the men are largely incapable of performing these caring task (Dworzanowski-Venter, 2008; Dworzanowski-Venter & Smith, 2008).

4 The continued relevance of HIV and AIDS activism

"Help prevent a sequel" ...[1]

Introduction

In the previous chapter, we have seen the manner in which configurations around HIV and AIDS gave rise to claiming new forms of citizenship albeit fraught with insecurities and other complex "glocal" contingencies. The participation in activism is equally vested in manifestations of citizenship as well as in processes of heightened democratization as it leads to alternative forms of knowledge generation and the unlocking of opportunities previously not conceivable in the public sphere (Jungar & Oinas, 2010). Although patient involvement and advocacy in health sciences did exist before the onset of AIDS, this disease's activism managed to venture into (from relatively early on) the well-guarded worlds of scientific knowledge production and accompanying health policy development (Epstein, 1996). However, it is the specific manifestation of informed and political activism or *trendy activism* that has grabbed the world's attention in unprecedented ways and not necessarily the more mundane, less spectacular, and largely overlooked appearances of activism that persisted and still somehow continue to persist (Burchardt, 2014).[2] Scholars tend to ignore those HIV and AIDS responses that are not high in profile although they might be more prevalent within communities (Chazan, 2008). The emphasis on a specific type of HIV activism, highly visible, and politically engaged is vested in the exceptional character it has obtained from the early years of the AIDS epidemic. Remarkable and trendy AIDS activism stretches from the early years, when the US-based Act Up activist group first started pushing its cause of access to AIDS treatment, up until the more recent manifestations of visible and political activism in the global South, the Treatment Action Campaign (TAC) being the *cause célèbre* in this context.

Despite the resemblance of South African AIDS activism to forms of activism that was garnered against the apartheid state, current HIV advocacy has managed to carve itself a unique and recognizable path in the political and social imagination (locally and globally) and has been studied rather intensely. In fact, HIV activism in South Africa, especially advocacy performed by the well-known and amply researched TAC, is widely lauded as an exemplary and successful social movement, one characterized by its grassroots mobilization or "globalization from below" (Appadurai, 2001). It is, therefore, now widely acknowledged that similar processes of "lay expertification" (Epstein, 1996) and "citizen science" (Irwin, 1995) – concepts used to explain the increase in ordinary citizens' actions to mitigate the flawed official response to a range of dangers, disease being but one – have equally taken on a unique form in post-apartheid South Africa. This is indicative of the manner in which the exceptional activist responses that have characterized HIV and AIDS from its onset have found fertile ground in South Africa albeit in circumstances that are so vastly different compared to where AIDS activism first took form.

The victories of HIV and AIDS activism are many and well known, and this focus is, therefore, not the aim of this chapter. This chapter rather focuses on contemplating the dangers associated with activism being framed as exceptional, on the one hand, and the manner in which South African HIV and AIDS activism has developed HIV and AIDS activism in order to *withstand* the erosion of this exceptionality, on the other.

The complex assemblages that HIV and AIDS gave rise to – activism probably being one of the most critical components characterizing the materialization of the disease's realities among significant numbers of ordinary people – have inevitably ushered in unprecedented political stakes globally but also in the South African context. HIV and AIDS has come to be equated to issues of governance and of government, of legitimacy, and of care. The political stakes were strikingly evident in the unfolding of the 2000 AIDS Conference, held for the first time on African soil in Durban, South Africa. South African activists worked ceaselessly and strategically to claim the legitimate space and voice for their exigencies in a time that marked very limited possibilities of antiretroviral therapy (ART) access. Ironically, this conference happened at the height of former president Thabo Mbeki's overt skepticism about the scientific explanations related to HIV and AIDS and his entanglement with so-called "dissident" HIV science and views.[3] The political stakes were evident with the rather theatrical demonstration of Mbeki's objections – walking out midway through a public, heart wrenching presentation at the conference by the then 11-year-old, HIV-positive Nkosi Johnson[4] (who died in June 2001), supplicating the South African government to make prevention-of-mother-to-child medication available to all. Mbeki's actions were in stark contrast to the message of unity and cooperation in the speech of the South African icon, the late president Nelson Mandela during the same historical conference. The Durban Conference is often considered a watershed moment in the global response to HIV and AIDS. The conference was imbued with the strong moral imperative of finding rapid solutions to the roll-out of ART to all those in need of them and not just to those residing in the global north (Grebe, 2011). This "moral imperative" – as discussed later in relation to the legitimacy of the TAC – was to a large extent fundamental to the many successes that the TAC enjoyed over the years.

This conference highlighted exceptionality within exceptionality: the exceptional international political currency that HIV held in those days was combined with the volatile political and epidemiological context of South Africa, still raw from the devastation of years of apartheid and readying itself for a new struggle over yet another issue of survival: HIV and AIDS. This time around, complicating the issue, the fight had to be fought against a legitimately elected government – a government with an enormous support-base among many ordinary South African citizens.

Could HIV and AIDS activism that has taken shape within such an exceptional context (not only internationally but more certainly within the borders of South Africa) be seen as a transformative force which turns those mostly affected by HIV into "global human rights advocates," engendering "active citizenship" (Jungar & Oinas, 2010)? This question becomes all the more complicated seeing that this exceptional activism took root within the context of state legitimacy and wide support for the state. This obviously rendered activism much more complicated compared to exercising activism against a racist and exclusionary government and government policies. The exceptionality, therefore, stretches to yet another level: HIV and AIDS activism in South Africa had to reinvent itself in order to navigate an entirely new struggle. However, I would argue that among AIDS activists in South Africa, the *reinvention of activism* was soon realized to be a non-negotiable aspect of taking HIV and AIDS advocacy to the next level. This reinvention of activism has allowed the TAC and its various allies to remain relevant even in contemporary times marked by normalization and growing biomedicalization. Today, activism is as indispensable as in the years that marked denialism and the global hesitancy to allow access to ART. However, contemporary activism has become much less sensational and riveting. This chapter will explain some aspects that continue to legitimize health advocacy in South Africa largely under the banner of the TAC.

The epochs of activism

It helps to situate HIV activism in a timeframe in order to understand the contemporary stakes and challenges. Several academic renditions have tried to make sense of activism by classifying it into specific periodizations. Powers (2017), in a similar vein to feminist theory, translates HIV activism in South Africa to first- and second-wave activism. The first wave, he suggests, corresponds to activism that characterized those movements that stood up against state violence in the late-apartheid era. It was through the establishment of "social justice-oriented legal organizations" because of events such as the Soweto Uprising in 1976 and the death in detention of the famous Black Consciousness leader, Steven Bantu Biko, in 1977 that this activism first took off. The creation of activist organizations paved the way for first-wave HIV activist movements to emerge, largely driven by "white, gay, male and professional" activists (Powers, 2017). Second-wave activism, as developed by Powers (2017), was marked by "demographic shifts" to the "poor and working class" and a "change in the tactics utilized" (for example, making use of a civil disobedience campaign). This was done in order to make access to lifesaving ART available to those infected with HIV and dying of AIDS. In the main, this second wave was led by the TAC and the AIDS Law Project (ALP) and can be traced to the period just after the AIDS-related death of the gay rights activist, Simon Nkoli, in November 1998.

Christopher Colvin (2014) – echoing an earlier article by Richard Parker (2011) – divides HIV and AIDS activism into roughly three epochs; his periodization focusing more on a transnational level. The first era corresponds to the initial identification of the dreadful disease among gay men in the global North which ushered in the race to develop effective treatment in response to HIV's appearance. The second timeline is associated with the quest to make ART available in those areas that came to be known as the worst affected areas globally, namely in the global South. The structural constraints of deficient health systems, generalized epidemics, and constrained resources steered activism into a direction that was intractably involved in wider issues of social justice and inequalities. Colvin (2014) is of the opinion that these first two phases were largely "framed and energized through the lens of crisis and emergency," and that this "urgent specter" is understandable in a context of "needless death and suffering." The third and current era is marked by an epoch in which past victories in relation to access to ART has to be sustained and further developed to accommodate ever-increasing numbers of people who are in need of this lifesaving treatment. New treatment regimens as well as biomedical prevention interventions form part of the current activist debates and "more diffuse and ambiguous notions" that characterize chronic conditions (Colvin, 2014) are largely replacing the urgency of the first two eras. A central line of argumentation that Colvin develops is that despite similarities between these three ideal-typical periods within AIDS activism, there are very distinctive political stakes as well as unique health system and epidemiological challenges that characterize each unique periodization. The current period's distinctive challenges are identified as having to negotiate the controversial issue of expanding ART programs at scale and into sustainable treatment and prevention responses in an environment plagued by diminishing global health funding where competing health demands are all appealing for funding attention, and where there is increasing attention to the protection of patent rights.[5] Moreover, challenges also relate to design, implement, manage, and evaluate "combination prevention efforts that work simultaneously at the biological, behavioral and structural scales" (Colvin, 2014). Colvin continues, with what is probably the most important issue that this chapter would like to highlight, that

> these efforts will require the development of new concepts and theoretical frameworks in the basic, clinical, and social sciences as well as *new activist strategies for mobilizing this evidence in ways that maintain the earlier eras' productive dialectics of research, practice, advocacy and policy*.
>
> (Colvin, 2014, emphasis added)

In addition, any social movement or campaign's success will be greatly influenced by the manner in which it avoids being confined to the margins. Attracting support and attention from powerful social groups and potential influential allies is essential in order to maintain the momentum of a social movement and even more so in conditions that are marked by increased normalization of the core issue that is addressed.

Pitfalls of exceptional activism

For obvious reasons, the normalization of a phenomenon such as a fatal disease is pursued. These obvious reasons are vested in two determining factors. First, normalization is often associated with biomedical interventions that translate into lifesaving or palliating results. Second, processes of normalization have the potential to render the "exceptional" more mundane and, one would imagine, therefore less stigmatized and stigmatizing. Exceptional medical conditions with very limited biomedical interventions often have the potential to develop into stigmatized conditions shrouded in myths and misperceptions. Normalization equally has the contradictory potential to "kill activism" as was indicated by some activists in the UK in a study done by Steven Robins who identified dwindling activism in light of the availability of ART and the largely sanitized discourse around HIV and AIDS in the UK (Robins, 2005). In the next section, I will compare the plight of a non-exceptional disease, tuberculosis (TB) with an exceptional one, HIV. This is to indicate the potential trajectory that a non-exceptionalized HIV might take in the near future. Thereafter, I will highlight instances of activism, in the name of HIV and AIDS, that inadvertently jeopardize what activists set out to do in the first place: to secure responsible and sustainable access to everyone in need of ART. This section of the chapter indicates the intense difficulty to manage demands of ever-increasing health needs in a world marked by persistent and growing inequalities and the minefield of ethical considerations and interpretations in this environment of continued research and monitoring that marks biomedical normalization.

Something as simple as the treatable, yet deadly disease: TB

Comparing an exceptional disease like HIV and AIDS with a contemporary non-exceptional[6] one, *Mycobacterium tuberculosis* (TB) – also labeled "the forgotten plague" (Farmer, 2000) – indicates to what extent exceptionalization worked toward attaining levels of attention to HIV that had never been witnessed in the case of TB. This is the case despite TB being seen in the late 19th century as a disease with the potential to destroy European civilization (Ryan, 1993, in Farmer, 2000). TB or "Consumption" is undeniably a disease of poverty as its ravages are globally evident according to stratification previously called "differential susceptibility." Moreover, it has been noted that the "advent of effective therapy [as from 1943] seems only to have further entrenched this striking variation in disease distribution and outcomes" as the simplicity of TB treatment has simply not translated into sustained and enhanced treatment outcomes among those most affected and who often are the poor.

In a context of normalization, where I specifically refer to widespread complacency, the pitfalls of exceptionality are squarely in line with lessons learnt in the past when diseases were simply not branded with an exceptional label. In South Africa, as is the case globally, TB (which today is the top killer in South Africa) never enjoyed the potent mix of contextual factors that somehow converged exceptional activism with scientific and political vigilance and reaction to respond to its materialization. TB did have its own heyday, as was witnessed with the creation of the International Tuberculosis Campaign (ITC) which was the first coordinated effort to globally control the disease that affected so many people and was heralded "the greatest medical crusade in history" by the *New York Times* in 1948 (Packard, 2016). In 1993, the World Health Organization (WHO) labeled TB a "global emergency," and a global DOTS (directly observed therapy short course) campaign was called for in order to respond to this problem (Dixon & Tameris, 2018). The critique of this "static response" to TB has been amply recorded, especially by anthropologists who have indicated the flaws associated with a narrow focus of DOTS on individual adherence. This focus happened at the expense of incorporating analyses that are cognizant of the structural forces and structural violence that undermine patient adherence. Such renditions, it is argued, will provide a more complex and nuanced rendition of being afflicted with TB in light of the new afflictions of M-DR and X-DR TB infections (Farmer, 2000; Harper, 2006).

In South Africa, M-DR TB has a higher mortality than the "new kid-on-the-block" disease, Ebola. However, the "amount of programmatic and political attention pales against a disease not seen in South Africa since 1995, but which commands resources and focus across the country" (Venter, 2016).[7] Even a seemingly convincing plan by the former minister of Health, Dr Aaron Motsoaledi, to have a unique TB 90-90-90 program (similar to the ambitious WHO plan) has not resulted in an "exceptional" status to befall TB. Nor former president Nelson Mandela's impassioned plea during the 2004 AIDS conference in Bangkok where he astutely stated that "we can't fight AIDS unless we do much more to fight TB as well" seemed to provide the right "mix" of factors to develop an exceptional TB action.

Dr Francois Venter (2016) indicates the need to have a similar combination of "energy, creativity, and most importantly, budget that the HIV world has enjoyed for over a decade." "Budget" is indeed a massive factor, considering that for every US dollar spent of HIV research; a meager US$0.05 is spent on TB research (Harrington, 2010). The HIV market is estimated to be worth approximately US$8 billion per year compared to a TB market of less than US$6 million a year. It is also revealing that no new class of drugs to treat TB has been approved since the 1960s which renders TB, in the words of Mark Harrington (2010), the "ultimate neglected tropical disease."

It is hard to believe that more people than ever before is living with a disease, "older than history" (Harrington, 2010). *Mycobacterium tuberculosis* (TB)'s resurgence in the 1990s,[8] after some years of containment, is a sinister omen of the manner in which the much younger HIV pathogen might be responded to in the near future. Harrington (2010) portends,

> One lesson from the history of TB that is pertinent to the struggle against AIDS is that a spate of early victories in TB control – the discovery of the organism through and diagnosis with acid-fast sputum smear micros-copy and culture, vaccination with bacilli Calmette-Guérin (1921) and chemotherapy (1948–1986) – led to complacency and decades of neglect. During this period, the field of TB science became drained of financing, skipping a whole generation of scientists (...).

By the 1950s, the world was convinced that TB was well on its way to being eradicated, which led to a complete cessation of trying to tackle the disease at its root causes. This rings alarm bells for a world which proclaims the "end of AIDS" and the ambitious UNAIDS 90:90:90 goals. The rise of TB drug resistance was produced by the failure of health systems all over the world to adequately and consistently treat those afflicted with TB (Packard, 2016).

HIV treatment development and research were egged on by vocal activists who demanded the use of inadequate and immature surrogate markers. This, in turn, led to speeding up processes of drug development immensely. These endeavors, steeped in urgency, invited more drug companies to join the ex-citing race of novel discoveries associated with drug combinations, which ultimately led to the effective triple-therapy regimens in 1996 (Harrington, 2010). Mark Harrington (2010) rightfully speculates as to the consequences of using these surrogate markers in ascertaining "anti-TB drug activity in real time, rather than requiring long-term trials of hundreds or thousands of patients with clinical end-points of relapse, reinfection, or death." He too indicates that despite more than 125 years of research on TB, "there is still far too little information about its *in vivo* pathogenesis inside the human body," as well as a dearth of understanding of TB genetics compared to that of HIV.[9] This is again testimony to the immense action by AIDS advocacy, especially in the global North but with concrete results all over the globe.

Activism and the ethics of social and biomedical research

South African AIDS exceptionality was largely the result of a specific global socioeconomic and political alignment in which AIDS first appeared (and developed into a treatable condition). For example, the confluence of the end of apartheid with the sharp rise in HIV infections could potentially serve to justify the "tolerance" and interest in the topic of "AIDS denialism." Under different circumstances, most individuals (all the more with the status of pres-ident) uttering such dangerous, callous, and farfetched ideas about the etiology of HIV would probably be summarily dismissed and ostracized. However, the unique history of South Africa's recent past, in combination with the climbing prevalence of HIV, made for a compelling and fascinating narrative. Didier Fassin's 2007 monograph, *When bodies remember. Experiences and Politics of AIDS in South Africa*, is a case in point. In fact, in a review of this book, South African academic and author, Jonny Steinberg questions this tolerance toward the dissident (and deleterious) Mbeki stance (although convincingly and strongly articulated by Fassin), calling it "an anthropology of low expectations" (Steinberg, 2007). The denialism phase and the accompanying proliferation of quackery (Geffen, 2010) were indirectly engendered by the culmination of the tragic consequences of years of racism, oppression, and undermining and vilifying black African South Africans. These "denialist" years provided activists, academics, and critics with a lot of food for thought and also unleashed a host of social scientific enquiries that tried to somehow make sense of HIV through the specter of a very specific historical lens. This period equally pried open an unprecedented opportunity for AIDS activists to prove their worth by responding ethically in the face of the pernicious phenomenon of widespread AIDS dissidence. Given the proliferation of HIV activities around the globe, and the currency it has in terms of asking wider questions related to ethics in the research sphere, HIV has opened up a space to contest and question certain practices as well as representations beyond mere biomedical ethics. This was evident by the reflexive accounts that AIDS in the aftermath of apartheid gave rise to, such as accounts that took seriously the reasons behind South African AIDS denialism despite its devastating consequences.

In fact, AIDS, exceptionality vested in the sacrosanct notion of human rights, has unleashed a moral high ground for those involved in activism. However, this exceptional right to question practices in the process of trying to develop more efficient or more affordable care regimens is not necessarily shared by all activists (Geffen & Gonsalves, 2008). In the article by Nathan Geffen and Gregg Gonsalves (2008), it becomes clear how activists, easily united around the simple issue of access, could diverge rather radically when it comes to researching the feasibility and affordability of access at scale. Activism in times of normalization becomes more complex and fragmented where the division between "right" and "wrong" is not that visibly evident as during the exceptional years of blatant treatment denial.

Act-Up Paris is a revered activist group and one of the oldest in AIDS activism. This group questioned some research projects conducted to optimize ART in contexts where many people need to access it, and where resources are rather limited. This activist group caused the discontinuation of Tenofovir trials in 2004–2005, which tested the efficacy of pre-exposure prophylaxis. In 2006, Act-Up Paris also objected to the DART trial that studied whether ART could be administered without routine laboratory testing and whether patients could undergo structured treatment interruptions. The factors studied during these trails are obviously important to consider in light of the ever-growing need to get people onto ART in contexts of severe health system failure as well as constrained resources. Another activist group, the Dutch group SOMO (*Stichting Onderzoek Multinationale Ondernemingen*), also published a briefing of what they labeled "unethical trials," which equally included the Tenofovir and DART trials already alluded to, as well as the HIVNET 012 trial that took place in Uganda to test the efficacy of single-dose Nevirapine to reduce the risk of mother-to-child transmission (MTCT) of HIV. The accusations related to the latter trial were largely based on erroneous media reporting of serious irregularities within the study and SOMO even compared the trial to the disreputable Tuskegee experiment (a hallmark example of gross ethical negligence). The controversy around the HIVNET 012 trial fueled pseudo-scientists to continue denying the link between HIV and AIDS and to undermine the option of availing Nevirapine in South Africa and elsewhere (Geffen & Gonsalves, 2008). Act-Up Paris, together with some other organizations, also attempted to derail a circumcision intervention in Orange Farm, Johannesburg, and during a 2007 conference on women and AIDS in Nairobi, one of the members of Act Up also accused panel members discussing the findings of the Nonoxynol-9 trial of "killing 900 women" during this research.[10] Nathan Geffen and Gregg Gonsalves (2008) wrote an article denouncing this "irrational" activism as dangerous precedents in the continued and sustained fight against HIV and AIDS. Although all examples that were cited could be defective on bioethical grounds, contextual factors render these trials important in sustaining the ART response globally. In fact, ethically complex interventions seldom harbor "right" or "wrong" answers but require consistent and rational justifications of opting (or not) for some actions. The ethical argumentations as to the objections of these trial studies surely do hold merit at first glance, but ethical deliberations, and especially the tension of utilitarianism versus individual rights, are very tangible in these examples, and at times, some of the accusations were just plainly bizarre and false. Navigating the right form of activism has in itself become a complex task within the AIDS industry. Geffen and Gonsalves (2008) indicate that too often, "ideology has trumped science" in the quest to deliver treatment at scale. AIDS activism is well known for its moral high ground, and unfortunately, this moral high ground is often juxtaposed with the term coined by Jon Cohen (2006) of "pharmanoia" which simply means an irrational suspicion of pharmaceutical companies, their research, and their products. "Pharmanoia," the *enfant terrible* within the family of AIDS activists, is a dangerous precedent because of the "rights discourses" that have come to shape the AIDS landscape as well as the AIDS research landscape. Jon Cohen (2006) rightly points out that

> AIDS has ushered in an ethos in which more and more people, especially in desperately poor countries, want to know what's in it for them to participate in a clinical trial. The want some say in establishing what researchers call the risk/ benefit ratio. These are reasonable demands. But pharmanoia makes them harder to hear.

Moreover, the so-called "unethical" trials all happened in the developing world, mostly in Africa, where an acute sensitivity still prevails given the historical legacy of equating AIDS with Africa, with backwardness, and with sexual prowess, as indicated in Chapter 2. Decrying ethical breaches has so much more currency in this context.

The differences in opinions as to the "ethical" manner in which services around HIV treatment should be researched is also indicative of the different geopolitical realities of countries faced with stark differences in prevalence and resources. Even purported ethically fool proof interventions, such as the "test and treat" approach[11] for pregnant mothers to prevent MTCT and to reduce maternal deaths, rolled-out in Malawi, raised plenty of questions around the ethics of such an intervention (Colvin, 2014). Some of the ethical issues that were raised included differences in treatment access (prioritizing pregnant women), the long-term effects of starting treatment at such an early stage, the effects of this program on other patients seeking treatment in the context of a constrained health system, issues of adherence and resistance, the neglect of other health needs in light of such an aggressive ART intervention, etc. (Coutsoudis et al., 2013 in Colvin, 2014). A scientific storm also raged over the uncertain outcomes after subsequent trails to test the use of second-generation microbicides[12] as a form of pre-exposure prophylaxis among women. When scientific evidence from the FEM-PrEP and VOICE trials failed to back the positive trial results of the 2010 CAPRISA 004 microbicide trial results, the activist community, who was pushing to fast-track the roll-out of the microbicide based on the results of the CAPRISA 004 trial, was totally taken aback. In fact, the speed at which activists demanded the interpretation of results as well as exerting pressure for the treatment to become available to women was described as "politically and scientifically expedient" (Montgomery, 2015). It is, however, resonant with the manner in which AIDS research was fast-tracked in the past when activists were prepared to take risks if only it could lead to faster access to treatment options to prevent infections or to treat the disease.

The ethical terrain of HIV and AIDS is all the more tricky to navigate in the midst of the unique confluence of a rampant HIV and AIDS epidemic within a historical context where a fledgling democracy had to make sense of a deadly disease striking at the heart of its constituency. The unprecedented context of HIV and AIDS activism within South Africa has rendered this group of activists vulnerable to many accusations: being "unpatriotic," "anti-African," and lackeys of the international pharmaceutical companies (Robins, 2004). It was even said that some senior government politicians

> in an attempt to discredit the TAC, claim that its leadership, in particular Zachy Achmat,[13] had a "hidden agenda," which was to introduce "liberal" ideas about sexuality that are in line with those held by the international gay and lesbian movement.
>
> (Robins, 2004)

The former minister of health, the late Manto Tshabalala-Msimang, also accused Mark Heywood of being a "white man" manipulating black people. She said that people

> come with busses and go to commissions where they wait for the white man to tell them what to do ... Our Africans say: Let us wait for the white man to deploy us; to say to us: *toyi-toyi* (protest) here.
>
> (in Friedman & Mottiar, 2004)

The TAC was first part of the National Association with People living with AIDS (NAPWA) but the relationship soon ended after initial disagreements about political strategies and tactics (Mbali, 2013). This relationship soured even further and became openly hostile after the TAC accused NAPWA of dishonest and corrupt dealings. This initial division within the activist ranks led to acrimonious exchanges between the two groups, with NAPWA also gaining the support of former minister Tshabalala-Msimang.

In contexts where the "signification" of disease (Treichler, 1987) has such enormous traction, "conversion to 'mainstream' AIDS science may be partial and precarious" (Robins, 2004). "Religious, spiritual and 'traditional' explanations and modes of healing are significant contenders in the struggle to fight and make sense of HIV/AIDS" (Robins, 2004). On the other hand, biomedicalization and normalization of ART also lead to entrenching some undesired consequences that cast ethical shadows as to its deployment. Steven Robins (2004) refers to the conversation he had with a well-known figure in activist circles, Dr Eric Goemaere, an influential figure and *Médecins Sans Frontières* doctor who worked in some of the earliest ART roll-out programs in South Africa. He indicated the "Janus-like character" of ART and of other biomedical technologies,

> Goemaere pointed out that whereas ART can undoubtedly prolong lives, it can also become a conduit for the "medicalization of poverty" and the creation of dependencies on medical experts and drugs. Although MSF consciously seeks to counter disempowering and normalizing biomedical discourses by stressing citizen rights to health care and medical and scientific knowledge, such messages are seldom heard in the public health clinics. Instead, clinic nurses and doctors tend to reproduce hierarchical and paternalistic expert-patient relations.
>
> (Robins, 2004)

Activism, and claiming the moral high ground within the assemblages of the HIV and AIDS world, is fraught with tensions. It stretches beyond mere bioethical norms that normally (and often too mechanistically) characterize medical trials and interventions. Taking an activist stance and making claims in the field of HIV and AIDS are steeped in the historic and the present moral economies of a wide variety of stakeholders in the AIDS industry.

The TAC in South Africa and the "politics of morality"

After the official downfall of apartheid in 1994, many leaders of civic organizations and nongovernmental organizations (NGOs) were canvassed to fill powerful leadership positions within regional and national government structures. In this climate of legitimacy and democracy, these NGOs and civic organizations that had previously been oppositional forces of government were now increasingly aligning themselves with the newly elected governmental powers (Mindry, 2008). Inevitably, this rapprochement with government, the shared vision, and partial financing by the state led to a new set of tensions. The alliance greatly complicated the monitoring role that such organizations normally should undertake *vis-à-vis* the ruling government. An example of one of these early post-apartheid developments was the case of the implementation of the Reconstruction and Development Program (RDP) that came into existence in the early 1990s in order to remedy past injustices in access to basic human needs, privations that were exacerbated during many years of racial discrimination. The RDP advanced an approach of "bottom-up transformation" but simultaneously required the state to perform this plan in a "top-down manner" in order to ensure its implementation. This was but one example where NGOs and civic organizations developed a close relationship to the state while performing their monitoring role. It was also in this context of the early 1990s when "discourses on empowerment shift[ed] the focus away from social problems towards a neoliberal emphasis on individual actualization through self-management" (Mindry, 2008).

Despite this moment of seeming harmony between the state and civic organizations, AIDS activism, largely under the banner of the TAC,[14] still managed to capitalize on what Sidney Tarrow (1994) calls a "political opportunity structure." A unique confluence of circumstances gave rise to AIDS activism in South Africa in the post-apartheid context. There is a dearth of renditions tracing the rise of this extraordinary civic movement within a historical background to indicate how AIDS activism entered the political realm with such authority and thereby becoming a dominant force in the AIDS landscape. Some accounts do deal with the important historic precedent that left an indelible mark on the development of AIDS activism in South Africa (Robins, 2004; Friedman & Mottiar, 2005; Grebe, 2011; Mbali, 2013; Powers, 2017). Theodore Powers (2017) indicates that initial AIDS activism in South Africa not only focused on "horizontal" or transnational ties led to the immense successes of this movement. Powers (2017) indicates that through activists' understanding of the "vertical" power of activism in other words "continuities" with older forms of local activism, they ensured the strengthening of much-needed legitimacy that subsequently characterized this lobby group's long-term survival despite a variety of onslaughts (as seen earlier). This vertical approach puts a high premium on "interpersonal ties of South African HIV and AIDS activists that carried across historical time" and this approach describes how "inter-personal networks transmit knowledge and/or knowledge practices across time" (Latour, 2005 in Powers, 2017). Zachy Achmat also indicates, in an interview with Eduard Grebe (2011), the importance of "institutional memory of activism."[15] Equally, the strong international ties rendered the TAC's struggle more visible and justifiable in the eyes of very important allies, such as the global media as well as the influential scientific community. The importance of embarking on a global campaign was identified as an indispensable element within the South African fight for ART, according to Zachy Achmat (in Grebe, 2011). These alliances led to the conducive environment that set the scene for global victories. One such victory was the November 2001 Doha Declaration which added the important clause to the TRIPS (Trade Related Intellectual Property Rights) agreement (as already alluded to). This clause stated that developing countries, when faced with public health crises, do not necessarily have to adhere to the intellectual rights associated with pharmaceutical products as would normally be the case. The development and importation of generic medicines therefore, became possible to exercise legally.[16] In Grebe's article (2011), he indicates that Zachy Achmat ascribed the ratification of the Doha Declaration not only to the leading role played by the Brazilian government and *Médecins Sans Frontières*' international campaign but also to the watershed Pharmaceutical Manufacturers Association (PMA)[17] case that took place in South Africa. According to Achmat, this case established the engrained link between intellectual property rights, on the one hand, and access to ART, on the other.

The moment was propitious for AIDS activism to take root in the South African context largely because of the international milieu of growing advocacy, support, and interest in the disease (as elucidated in Chapter 2) but also because of the internal configuration of events which encouraged collective action in the aftermath of the gains against an oppressive state apparatus. Moreover, Zachy Achmat argued that the TAC's principal source of strength was the fact that it mobilized a strategic resource or element necessary for successful activism. This strategic resource was the creation of a "moral consensus" among its heterogeneous supporters, and this element[18] was entrenched in the face of perceived weaknesses of morality on the part of government in tackling issues around HIV (not discrediting the entirety of the state, as opposition politics might be tempted to do; Friedman & Mottiar, 2004). Grebe (2011) also describes the rights-based approach taken by the TAC as indicative of the "politics of moral consensus" that was subscribed to by the TAC. He specifically refers to the use of litigation to bring to fruition those legal rights explicitly developed within the South African Constitution post-apartheid. Grebe (2011) is of the opinion that

> By frequently stating that the rights it insists upon are guaranteed by the Constitution, it both strengthens the moral force of its appeal by locating it within the trajectory of South Africa's liberation and makes clear that its challenge is not to the legitimacy of the government or the state, but to government policies.

Morality might have been the glue that kept AIDS activism intact, but according to the prominent South African scientist, Professor Hoosen Goovadia, "the denialist attacks on science and evidence-based health policy did more to politicize [our] thinking than the moral claims around treatment access" (interview with Goovadia in 2008 in Grebe, 2011). It would be interesting to explore the affinity that science entertains with activism today in a context of widespread normalization through the generalized access to ART. Grebe (2011) grasps this paradox in South African AIDS activism that also foreshadowed current predicaments inasmuch as the end of AIDS denialism removed a source of *powerful public support and attention* from the TAC. One can even venture into saying it removed a level of melodrama, given the unprecedented and unthinkable actions that accompanied AIDS denialism which had to be fought and contested by activists as is depicted in the detailed account of Nathan Geffen (2010) on AIDS dissent and accompanying charlatanism and opportunism. It now leaves AIDS activism to deal with mundane issues of bureaucratization in a climate of widespread normalization.

The morality associated with these activists is indicative of yet another layer of "exceptional morality" (as highlighted in Chapter 2) albeit in a positive sense and not in the judgmental manner that suffused issues of HIV and AIDS. It would have seemed inconceivable for the African National Congress (ANC) government to be tarnished so soon after the end of apartheid's rule. However, the strategies deployed by the HIV activists somehow accommodated the multifarious and often contradictory politics of the post-apartheid South African state in moral and ethical ways, carefully toeing the line between respect and discord. In an interview in the early 2000s, Zachy Achmat indicated that the TAC wanted to get medicine to people and did not want to "cause a revolution" (in Friedman & Mottiar, 2004). In those early days of fighting for treatment, the TAC was often criticized by other social movement activists for not focusing its campaign on the government's then controversial macro-economic policy. The adoption of the neoliberal approach of the GEAR (Growth, Economic, and Redistribution) strategy, dubbed South Africa's self-imposed structural adjustment program, was seen by many as a step in the wrong direction when it came to redressing past issues and inequalities left by the legacy of years of discrimination (Bond, 2000; Cheru, 2001; Marais, 2001). Mark Heywood, one of the founders of the TAC, however, explained that their initiative in the year 2000 to import generic drugs for the treatment of HIV and AIDS was in itself addressing a structural issue and not merely one of simple access (Friedman & Mottiar, 2004). This delicate balance between overt and absolute confrontation and single-issue disputes marked the difficult early years of balancing support with dissent between a legitimate state, on the one hand, and an activist group that had in mind long-term relevance, on the other.

In the exceptional case of HIV and AIDS, social and political agendas were set in place firmly before the basic scientific facts of the epidemic were known (Scheper-Hughes, 1994). It has already been mentioned how Nancy Scheper-Hughes (1994) indicates the exceptionality of the AIDS epidemic because of it initially being framed as a crisis in human rights with obvious public health ramifications instead of it being a crisis in public health with important human rights components. The novelty of this focus – on rights and not on the disease *per se* – disregarded classic responses of public health. The TAC used the new constitutional armamentarium to activate rights-based provisions within this progressive document.[19] However, such a "rationalist and liberal individualist conceptions of the modern citizen as a rights-bearing subject are inadequate for understanding the transformative character" that new biosocial identities linked to HIV and AIDS and its activities ushered in. Stephen Robins (2005) is of the opinion that simply providing information and education about rights and responsibilities is not sufficient for creating what he calls, this "responsibilized citizen" (Robins, 2005). The notion of the "responsibilized citizen" was an invention of progressive public health specialists and organizations such as *Médecins sans Frontières* to address the unique necessities to ensure patients taking ownership and control of their ART regime and its accompanying challenges. It was for this reasons that these social movements (the TAC and MSF) equipped patients with an array of skills to inculcate an emphasis "on both health rights and responsibilities" (Robins, 2005). As from the earliest MSF treatment programs, the emphasis was thus to grapple with "both biological disease and the social, cultural and psychological dynamics associated with stigmatized identities" (Robins, 2005).

Despite the narrow focus that HIV and AIDS activism might seem to encompass, in South Africa, this activism has always been about much more than merely ART access. In the past, this was evident given the multifarious battles that had to be fought in "courts and streets" (Robins, 2004), against multinational pharmaceutical giants but also against the newly elected South African government during the time of denialism, fighting stigma and discrimination but also problematic myths and quackery that still flourish in the midst of this potentially debilitating disease. Their actions stretched into domains as varied as influencing anti-discrimination laws, ensuring patient access to medicine and care, enhancing and innovating scientific thinking and processes, and addressing health system reform, winning in the "court of transnational public opinion" (Olesen, 2006).

The individualist and narrow framing of "responsibility" in the context of HIV is also challenged by shifting the attention away from prevention to treatment. The TAC, therefore, has challenged many (judgmental) influential discourses about HIV that got entrenched in public policy, in the media, as well as in academic literature. A lot of these discourses were solely focused on prevention which tend to convey messages of individual behavior change (Jungar & Oinas, 2011). The TAC raised HIV from being a simple matter of individual behavior to gain increasing influence as an issue to be dealt with at the political level (Jungar & Oinas, 2010). Their demands for healthcare and medication disturbed discourses that ascribed inevitable blameworthiness to those with HIV and that gave those who were not (yet) infected the responsibility to protect themselves from the infected. The TAC's campaign for continued access to medication, therefore, aims to strengthen civil society and to revitalize the wider political landscape of democracy.

Why did people join and support the TAC in such high numbers? Was it simply because of their HIV and AIDS status or was it because of deeper social justice convictions? Was the issue at stake the creation of what Manuel Castells, following in the footsteps of Alain Touraine coined "project identities" which are identities that produce and are equally produced by wider collective projects which have as its aim social change in response to inequities (Castells, 1997)? The TAC realized that community mobilization is essential in building advocacy around an issue such as HIV. However, navigating activism in a context of widespread precariousness is much more complicated. Robins and Von Lieres (2004) indicate this complex dilemma

> that while the legal status of the majority of the people is assured, their experience of citizenship is ambiguous. They often remain excluded from effective economic and political participation. If South Africa's new democracy speaks to anything, it is to the uneasy intertwining of democracy and marginalization.

Activism has the potential to create "new 'middle-level' institutions capabable of representing the demands of marginalized people to the state" (Robins & von Lieres, 2004). This was seen to have been at play in the deployment of community health workers (CHWs), as indicated in the previous chapter. According to Cohen and Rai (2000 in Robins and von Lieres, 2004), this new politics at play in contemporary South Africa is a "sophisticated refashioning of 1980s anti-apartheid activism" as it too uses "the courts and the media, as well as local and transnational advocacy networks, along with grassroots mobilization and skilfull negotiations with the state." There is also a resemblance to globally connected new social movements that have emerged in many parts of the world in recent years.

These beneficial networks are also strengthened by what Ahmad (2013) calls the TAC's wielding of "three dimensions of lawyering." This manifests in their use of advocacy through litigation, as well as through advocacy in stimulating progressive change. But more importantly, the TAC also uses their activism to enhance pedagogic processes. In addition to their advocacy work, the TAC is a vocal political movement (greatly because of their past allegiances to struggle groupings during the fight against apartheid); however, it does not openly support any political party and is, therefore, not a "party political movement" (Friedman & Mottiar, 2004).

The successes linked to TAC's actions are greatly ascribed to their grassroots mobilization which was activated by the array of campaigns to enhance treatment literacy and awareness among people within schools, community centers, clinics, churches, and other areas of socialization. Joining the ranks of the TAC could be ascribed to a variety of factors, the two most prominent issues being that so many people's lives have been and still are affected by the disease and its ramifications but, second, also because of the social causes that undergird the functioning of the TAC. Friedman and Mottiar (2004) presciently pointed out the immense importance to allow for these two divergent rationales to co-survive within an organization such as the TAC, "ensuring that the gap between them does not create destructive tensions."

The organization places a premium on transparency and accountability, and openly avoids instances where conflicts of interest might jeopardize their image. Funding is, therefore, not necessarily accepted – in the past it did, not accept funding from the South African government nor from pharmaceutical companies. Even a funding body such as UNAIDS was deemed too entwined in the narrow interests of the US government (Friedman & Mottiar, 2004).

It was indicated that the TAC managed to straddle the difficult zones of cooperation and contestation with the new government post-1994. They have been involved in "creating a new post-apartheid politics of strategic engagement, partnership and negotiation," developing a "situationally framed politics shaped by shifting social and political realities" (Robins & von Lieres, 2004). Their political and legal strategies proved to stretch beyond simplistic binaries of "us" versus "them" to accommodate a politics of contingency. Striking unprecedented alliances, wielding significant symbolism, and raising larger issues of citizenship, albeit health citizenship in post-apartheid South Africa, have to a large extent provided this group with a legitimate voice. This approach, I will argue, is the only viable form of activism to confront most issues in the context of current South African politics and beyond. The TAC espouses secular and scientific approaches to explaining HIV and AIDS.

The TAC also managed to unsettle imbedded neoliberal perceptions of "agency." This they did not only by locating it in the larger collective but has done so by redefining the meanings of victimization. TAC activists are of the opinion that "prevention and treatment of HIV and AIDS are two sides of the same coin; similarly, they show that the victim and agent positions are also interconnected" (Jungar & Oinas, 2011). The TAC has, to a great extent, focused on the "middle ground of social practice" and not confined itself to either a simplified agentic stance nor an overly deterministic structural approach to dealing with HIV and AIDS issues (Kippax et al., 2013).

Their success has also been ascribed to the fact that an influential organization, such as the TAC, managed to transition rather smoothly from the earlier days characterized by them being a "small and highly flexible activist grouping held together by trust and a strong commitment to common goals, to a formal and bureaucratized organization that nevertheless retains many characteristics of the former" (Grebe, 2011). Grebe (2011) foresees that the TAC will run into difficulty if it tries to "incorporate the strengths of both 'activist movement' and 'corporate NGO' leadership models." He is of the opinion that the previously influential group Act Up in the United States failed to make this transition from "activist group" to "corporate NGO" which led to the weakening of their stature.

Conclusion

> The vibrancy of 2000 is no more. It has been replaced by calm and
> rational options for the future of the HIV epidemic made possible by a
> combination of scientific discovery, innovative funding mechanisms, and
> deep commitments from policy makers, activists, researchers, health care
> providers, and many others to make AIDS treatment available.
>
> (Abdool Karim & Abdool Karim, 2016)

The end of AIDS exceptionalism inevitably also reaches into the workings
and representations of activist groups all around the globe. Sustaining the
enormous impact of activism, as it has been manifesting for some years now,
is no mean feat. The widespread and successful national ART program is
extending normalizing biomedical discourses into the public discourse. This
has the increasing potential to result in citizens becoming passive consum-
ers of biomedical technologies and entrenching rational believes in scientific
expertise. Dr Francois Venter (2016) rightly points out that many problems
(and solutions) that we ascribe to the HIV and AIDS epidemic are, in fact,
not specific to HIV. In an optimistic view, refreshing in the current context
of cynicism that prevails normalization, he notes that

> HIV has allowed the whole area of health to be ambitious again, recon-
> necting with the energy that briefly arose after the Alma Ata declaration
> on primary health care, but perhaps with more critical reflection (and
> resources to support it). It is an exciting time to be in the health field,
> especially in HIV, and people in South Africa rely on us to get it right.

"Getting it right" often happened because of the tireless work of activists,
and as was witnessed in the continued necessity for activism, their continued advocacy will probably persist for some time to come. The manner in
which activism played a role in "speaking truth to power" globally and very
manifestly in South Africa should foreshadow the only sustainable solution to
true democratization in our globalized world. In South Africa, our current
political climate is in dire need of unflinching activism in order to retali-
ate against the continued untoward actions that happen under the banner of
governments all over the world. HIV and AIDS exceptionality crystallized
greatly because of the vibrancy and innovation of global and local forms of
activism. It is one example of exceptionality that should be marshaled to
continue the various struggles not only around access to better healthcare
but also to an array of other issues that could contribute to the eradication of
gaping inequalities in so many facets of everyday life.

The continued relevance of activism should balance universalist biomedical notions that underpin the specific manifestations of disease within a
context such as South Africa where alternative explanations of illness will
often vie for attention, provided the ubiquitous context of depravity and

precariousness. However, activism should continue to act as a catalyst to develop notions associated with citizenship, moving beyond the confines of health citizenship *per se*. The manner in which activism in South Africa engendered the democratization of science and expertise should be continued and infiltrate all sectors of our society. Continued activism needs to occupy a "politics of the moral high ground" as was characteristic of the early years of the TAC's activities and continues to mark the organization, together with its multiple allies, to occupy a difficult terrain of contestations, cooperation, and relevance in a global and local context in dire need of such action.

This chapter and the preceding one aimed to indicate the manner in which AIDS exceptionalism has paved the way for unique opportunities to not only legitimately contest governments and official institutions globally and locally but has also led to the expression and manifestation of new variations of citizenship, of belonging, and of questioning power from the margins. Surely, there is a continuation with erstwhile "democratizing aspirations" (Comaroff & Comaroff, 1999) and parallels to former struggles waged in the name of representation and rights. The literature is firmly in place to attest to this historical event that is still ongoing in the contemporary AIDS industry. In fact, CHW activity as well as activism have evolved from their "AIDS origins" to morph into new forms of claim staking: both "movements" have somehow adapted their actions to still remain relevant despite the waning of AIDS exceptionalism. In a time of increased neoliberal framing of disease, activism and the creation of new cadres of work harbor some potential as to challenge its growing hegemony. Activism initiates the focus on solidarities across borders and the employment of "innovative need" to lead to the creation of "scattered hegemonies" (Grewal & Kaplan, 1994) that can increasingly hold to account the domineering master narratives that have come to characterize our globe. These processes are increasingly necessary, not only to respond to HIV and AIDS but also to so many other social ills that afflict our world at an ever-growing scale. This is also necessary because the normalization discourses and concomitant actions are not aligned to the suffering and daily hardships that HIV and AIDS continues to foreground.

Notes

1 This is the last line from the documentary *"Fire in the Blood"* that marks the slow and contentious trajectory of securing access to ART.
2 Burchardt (2014) specifically refers to the widespread phenomenon of what she calls "Christian activism" in relation to issues of HIV and AIDS and the manner in which faith-based activism or forms of collective organization that do not fall under the banner of NGO activities are often not considered from a "social movement perspective" and, therefore, not afforded a lot of (academic) attention.
3 The "Durban Declaration" was signed at this AIDS conference in Durban by scientists all over the world and published in the reputable scientific journal *Nature*. In this declaration, the signatories affirmed their scientific unanimity in relation to the etiology of AIDS that was questioned by the president of the time, Thabo Mbeki.

4 Despite the immense pathos that Nkosi Johnson's speech implored (and continues to implore) from the emotionally charged crowds at the Durban AIDS Conference, this performance equally stirs our ethical sensibilities as to the manner in which suffering also becomes a commodity in mediatized times. Images of suffering are used to appeal both emotionally and morally to global and local audiences but too often leads to information overload and desensitization (see Kleinman & Kleinman, 1997).

5 In October 2018, South Africa hosted the global WIPO Conference (World Intellectual Property Organization) titled *"Respect for Intellectual Property – Growing from the Tip of Africa."* Section 27 together with the "Fix The Patent Laws" campaign used this opportunity to highlight the anomalies of the South African intellectual property industry, where too many medicines, available at much cheaper prices in other developing countries, were out of reach of the large majority of South Africans because of the South African government's "excessive respect for IP" (Section 27, 2018).

6 Feldberg (1995) notes that in 1949, it was evident that another disease, polio, was getting preferential attention compared to TB. At 30/100,000 cases of polio compared with cases exceeding 90/100,000 of TB, and a threefold mortality rate of TB compared to polio, TB's devalued and non-exceptional status was evident.

7 The comparison between early responses to HIV and AIDS and those that marked the recent resurgence of the Ebola disease can be found in an article by Gonsalves and Staley (2014).

8 In sub-Saharan Africa, there was a fivefold increase in TB in the 1990s because of HIV. TB is not considered an opportunistic infection of HIV but rather a co-infection, as it has its own "deadly and lengthy course" (Harrington, 2010).

9 At the time of the article in 2010, Harrington indicates that there were only six complete *M tuberculosis* genome sequences compared to thousands of those of HIV.

10 For the full explanation of the accusations associated with each trial, see Geffen and Gonsalves (2008).

11 This approach provides immediate lifelong ART to those diagnosed with HIV regardless of CD4 count or clinical presentation.

12 It was a South African epidemiologist Zena Stein who, in 1990, published what would become the first call to develop a microbicide to prevent HIV infection in women. Her paper was titled "HIV Prevention. The need for methods women can use" in the *American Journal of Public Health* (Montgomery, 2015).

13 Zachy Achmat, one of the founders and probably the most charismatic leader of the TAC, moved on to create an organization known as *Ndifuna Ukwazi* (meaning "I want to know" but changed to the English appellation "Dare to Know" www.nu.org.za). His new organization engages trainee-activist "fellows" and partner NGOs and communities in a range of activities with an aim to build literacy and active engagement among ordinary citizens. This is done by offering assistance to the public in terms of technical legal, financial, and medical expertise. NU also aims to use the lessons learned in the AIDS response beyond HIV to respond to other pressing socioeconomic and political problems.

14 It is important to note that this chapter is focused on AIDS activism in general and not on the TAC and its history uniquely. However, AIDS activism in South Africa – especially given the academic literature generated around this issue, basically exclusively synonymizes AIDS activism in South Africa with the TAC. Their development, trajectory, and victories are not the focus of this chapter. The focus is on the manner in which AIDS activism, dominated by the evidence that has been generated on the TAC, has again uniquely responded to the local manifestation of AIDS. The history of the TAC is the history of spectacular AIDS activist successes. There is however, a dearth of accounts that look into

AIDS activism other than that of the TAC. The lack of these types of accounts probably indicates the immense necessity of activism to be *visible* in order to be deemed *successful*.

15 Another element in the development of AIDS activism that is often gleaned over is the TAC's initial link with the National Association of People Living with HIV/AIDS (NAPWA). Here I refer to the early tensions between the founders of the two organizations (notably between Mary Crewe and Peter Busse of NAPWA and Zachy Achmat and Mark Heywood of TAC) and the continued strained relations that marked later years between NAPWA and the TAC (see Grebe, 2011, for a fleeting reference to this history).

16 As an act of open deviance against the TRIPS agreement that was respected by the South African government despite the Medicine and Related Substances Act of 1997, Zachy Achmat in 1998 illegally brought 5,000 doses of generically produced fluconazole back to South Africa from Thailand. The generic version of this medication in Thailand costed $0.25 compared to the exorbitant cost of $18.10 in South Africa at the time (in Powers, 2017).

17 In 1998, the PMA sued the South African government of the late president Nelson Mandela because of their objection to the South Africa's Medicine and Related Substances Act of 1997, which would have allowed for the importation and/or manufacture of cheaper generic medicines in cases of public health emergencies. The TAC acted as *amicus curiae*. When the case appeared in court in 2001, it became a massive source of international interest and media coverage, resulting in an "avalanche of negative publicity" for the so-called "Big Pharma" industry (Barnard, 2002). It led to the PMA withdrawing their lawsuit in April 2001, deemed a tremendous victory to (especially) local activism.

18 Friedman and Mottiar (2004) emphasize the distinction between the use of morality as a once-off strategy, on the one hand, and morality being an integral component of the organization, on the other. Deploying morality as simply a strategy will not hold the same legitimacy compared to building morality into the proverbial DNA of an activist organization. This means that all aspects (and not just strategic actions) should be imbued with morality: the management of finances, the election of leaders, the manner in which members are treated, accountable and transparent governance, etc. This is why a social movement, such as the TAC, holds so much more promise for the future of democracy compared to the retaliatory contestations that mark conventional political party politics in South Africa.

19 The Bill of Rights in the South African constitution unequivocally states that water, housing, healthcare, and a clean environment are basic rights to be enjoyed by all citizens.

5 The AIDS industry

Entanglements, ethics, and the future of AIDS as we know it

In the preceding chapters, trajectories of rendering HIV and AIDS exceptional were highlighted by analyzing an array of germane contextual factors that somehow culminated into this global phenomenon and its local distinctions, the focus being especially on the crystallization thereof in the South African environment. In an era of significant normalization with increasing advances of and access to antiretroviral therapy (ART), potential pitfalls are lurking in imagining future endeavors related to HIV and AIDS. This biomedical normalization and its accompanying challenges particularly beg the question as to the continued relevance and potential contribution in the domain of social sciences research on HIV and AIDS. However, it has also been seen that this biomedical normalization transcends mere medicinal uses but gives rise to a diversity of "assemblages" and "derivatives" at play in the wider scope of the emergence and the entrenchment of exceptional HIV and AIDS.

It is (too) often reiterated, especially in the global North, that we are now living in an "AIDS aftermath" (Chambers, 2004) rightly because of the miraculous effects of effective ART to treat HIV and render it "manageable" (in the jargon of normalized biomedicine). In South Africa, however, as in contexts in other parts of the global South, it has been specified that we cannot "treat ourselves out of this epidemic."[1] The argument about AIDS exceptionality is not confined to the epidemic alone but is moreover vested in terms of *responses* to it. Many similarities could be drawn between AIDS and other afflictions that are increasingly characterizing our global world where inequalities are steadily growing despite substantial amounts of resources dedicated to act on theses ills. The manner in which those in power as well as academia respond to these emerging afflictions is more than often indicative of *global* moral economies and what has been referred to as the "differential valuation" of human life (Farmer, 2000). The fluctuation and entanglement of structural and agentic realities and experiences are in many instances similar in its twisted and nefarious consequences where people are left vulnerable and at the mercy of institutions that largely rationalize and de-individualize suffering individuals and their plight, so tellingly characteristic of neoliberal times and increasing market fundamentalism in which we are currently living. Suffering, especially *social* suffering – be it due to illness, displacement, natural disasters, famine, etc. – and the manner in which it is depicted, represented, responded to, and, ultimately, understood – revolves around the fact that this type of collective suffering "ruins the collective and the intersubjective connections of experience and gravely damages subjectivity" (Kleinman et al., 1997).

The issue of responding to societal ills becomes even more vexing in a paradoxical context where increasing assistance and interventions only seem to translate into ever-growing inequalities, thereby confining more and more human beings to the category of the indigent, the displaced, the homeless, the sick, the vulnerable, and the "at-risk." In the past, with access to tuberculosis (TB) medication, it was shown that the eventual availability of anti-tubercular treatment actually culminated into more unequal results in TB treatment outcomes – TB being the disease *par excellence* that is linked to poverty and differential valuing of people's lives. Does a similar fate await HIV and AIDS, as this epidemic too is tracking along "social fault lines" (Farmer, 1999). Will the normalization of HIV and AIDS culminate in the forewarnings of Max Weber that processes of institutionalization and accompanying standardization bring with it the increasing inability of critical purview, and this moreover in times of heightened feelings of AIDS disenchantment and lassitude? As with many other sensational topics, there is a limit on the valence of compassion and sympathy and an urgent need to "move on." The years of outrage witnessing preventable AIDS deaths are largely over (because of the efficacy of ART) although death because of AIDS is still a reality among so many groups and individuals who fall into the "at risk" (Nguyen & Peschard, 2003) conceptualizations all over the world, but more so in sub-Saharan Africa where new infections remain stubbornly high. In its wake, science moves on – where with HIV we are witnessing increased processes of progress translated into molecularization, technocratization, and the pharmaceuticalization of HIV. There is the urgent shift to quantify, to standardize, to control, and to attain levels of consistency and replicability within the domain of AIDS research and interventions. In such a context of unfettered progress and advances, the space for the unpredictable, the complex, and overlapping multifactorial contextual domains of behavioral, interpretative, social, and psychological aspects of this social disease is becoming increasingly problematic to justify and to sustain, being seen by many as becoming largely obsolete and anachronic. Drugs and its continued enhanced abilities it seems are after all epitomizing the "magic bullet" solution to the scourge despite warnings not to treat medication as such.

As indicated in the introductory chapter, there is often the notion of nostalgia that is reiterated by activists, researchers, and clinicians, when thinking back to the days when HIV had a more humane (and less molecular) face, when solidarity was simpler, and when the common enemy was the "three-letter plague" (Steinberg, 2008). Or perhaps this nostalgia is rooted in a more sinister sentiment, where certain stakeholders feel that the increased biomedicalization and technocratization of HIV is slowly portending the demise of their own careers, their professional livelihoods, and vested interests. Pisani (2008) levels criticism at the "ants in the sugar bowl" and "beltway bandits," who are attracted to partake in the AIDS response by the lure of increasing funding which too often resulted in organizations simply spending their budget rather than achieving tangible results.

As I indicated in Chapter 1, AIDS exceptionalism has wielded an unprecedented amount of resources in terms of funding, infrastructural development, capacity building, and employment opportunities, in both the medical and social research domains. This has often led us to perhaps being too engrossed in the politics of the moment. This preoccupation with the present is exactly what Jonny Steinberg critically reflects on in an article written in 2016. Bravely and eruditely (but certainly not nostalgically), he revisits his fieldwork notes that were generated during an ethnographic stint performed in the early years of ART availability (between 2005 and 2007) in a rural district in South Africa. In this article, he also questions the continued validity of the analysis of an ethnographic account of AIDS denialism by Didier Fassin (2007). He thereby arrives at a re-reading of his fieldwork notes by performing this critical reflexivity albeit retrospectively. This he does in today's context which is largely characterized by ART normalization and widespread acceptance, and he comes to the conclusion that his earlier focus was too steeped in the knowledge mold of the "denialist" time, and in an environment of historically rooted suspicion, as argued by Didier Fassin. In fact, this re-reading of his fieldwork notes and of Fassin's analysis allows him to "see" a new perspective among his participants (already present during the time of his fieldwork, but missed by him) of opportunity, anticipation, and hope that AIDS, HIV, ART, and the manifold interventions embryonically harbored as early on as in those early years of ART roll-out. He, therefore, questions and revises past interpretations not to discard or invalidate them but to somehow break the too often taken-for-granted categories and analyses that end up becoming master scripts of a disease that is ever-evolving within cacophonous contexts of local variabilities.

Issues of representation

> *It's all cliché, a communal sepia-toned memory that all us Aidsbabies have in common.*

(Lauren Beukes *Moxyland* 2008)

AIDS together with its all-encompassing research have inevitably given rise to the solidification of unique neologisms and appealing concept formations. New definitions have come to encapsulate the recurrence of concepts, such as the repeated usage of the term "marginality" which has been shown to indicate "to be positioned as the exception, the deviate, the parochial, *or the merely local in the face of the universal*" (Pigg, 2001, emphasis added). The recycling of ideas, building on them and differing from them – some strikingly similar to others – is indicative of the major investments at multiple levels to somehow contribute and partake in the once generous spoils of the AIDS industry. This recycling of ideas and the constant tinkering thereof also filtered down from academia and humanitarian interventions to reach those ordinary people whose lives are touched and acted on (or not) in a time of AIDS. Inevitably, it culminated into the creation of certain representations that greatly influenced and determined "the power to wound, to heal, or to prevent injury" (Nguyen & Peschard, 2003).

Georgina Feldberg (1995) indicates that dominant theories around TB from the mid-19th century onward gravitated toward "concern about differential susceptibility" and that these discourses dominated early understandings of TB, especially within the USA. These interpretations of "difference" depended to a great extent on the social perspectives of those making these claims, as "each generation attempted to make sense of this preferential, or differential, susceptibility, the explanations they offered reflected and reinforced their uncertainties about a changing scientific and social order" (Feldberg, 1995). Dorothy Nelkin (1995) opines that although scientific controversies and differences of opinion as to ways of acting in the face of disease typically revolve around issues that can be called "technical," these controversies – more often than not – are rather steeped in arguments about political and moral stakes. This was evident at a time of great uncertainty in the development and deployment of new ART access. In these early years, the ethical obligation to treat those in dire need was contrasted with the "zeitgest" of the time where emphasis was to focus on shielding the public from threats of diseases. It culminated into two distinct "regimes" of imagining global health (Lakoff, 2010). Those in favor of more generalized access to ART adhered to a view of global health in line with humanitiarian objectives as they saw in the AIDS epidemic and, in its consequences, the emergence of a medical disaster that needed to be addressed in order to respond to the accompanying human suffering. The other "regime of global health" constituted a view that was fixated on health security, with discourses pointing to the potential devastating consequences of drug-resistant HIV and the inability of health systems in the global South to cope with the general roll-out of ART. According to this regime of global health, the world had to be protected from this possible life-threatening scenario. The gist of this latter discourse was inherently political as it mostly revolved around issues of trust in the capacity of the ill in Africa to adhere to treatment regimes (McNeil, 2005).

Even in the face of evidence that directs pointedly to contrary findings to those of intervention expectations, discourses and regimes of knowing stubbornly persist and are sluggish to react to critique and alternative ways of thinking. It is expected that through social science research, especially through the in-depth engagement with people in their environments, that this realization (of unintended consequences or of failures), first enters the academic discourses. In earlier years of HIV and AIDS, Paul Farmer (1999) notes, for example, that it was rather surprising that "towards the end of the second decade of the AIDS pandemic, we still have no good evidence that primary prevention works." He is scathing of this extensive time lapse to lead to acknowledgment of this failure; a failure that cost tremendous amounts of money and resources because of the myriad global efforts that vociferously and religiously encouraged primary prevention. For him, "twenty years is a long time to wait for such candor," and his critique is even more disparaging as he opines that "one of the reasons for this delay is that the social scientists who might have offered critical assessments in a more timely fashion were too busy scrambling for their piece of the pie." The consequences of such excessive failures has a spillover effect, as Farmer cautions, that "we undermine faith in medicine and public health whenever we make unreasonable, excessive, or propagandistic claims" (Farmer, 1999). Despite the virtues of social sciences' views in light of the AIDS epidemic and its continued relevance, too often social scientists uncritically persist in blindly accepting and reinforcing ways of knowing. This inevitably leads to the proliferation of unsubstantiated claims, and the entrenchment of representations and practices that could have deleterious consequences and spillover effects for programs but more importantly, for people. It makes us, as social scientists, mere contributors or narrow specialists in the current "technocratic, problem-solving discourses" that "condition us to look outward from an expert's position, confident in the prospects of social engineering" (Scott, 1998 in Pigg, 2013).

We know that globally – even in the current times of generalized availability of ART and the immense promises inherent in this treatment – triage increasingly takes place, where only some places, some groups, and specific manifestations of disease are recognized by those determining the agenda of global health, while other groups and conditions fall by the wayside. This is an increasingly problematic ethical predicament identified by scholars, such as Betsey Brada (2013), and relevant to the conceptualization that encapsulates processes of exceptionalization and normalization in environments marked by precarious healthcare outcomes. Moreover, when this power (over life and death) is performed on seemingly unwitting and passive people, these very same people – through tactical strategizing of acceptance or resistance, and by expected and applauded acts of public performance – are constantly in a process to invent ways in which they could somehow fall (and remain) in categories of intervention and to avoid those of neglect or abandonment. The specific spirit or "zeitgeist" will be determining as to the manner in which subjectivity and temporality are enmeshed with each other (Mbembe, 2001) and will lead to ways in which people will buy into those markers that are "constituted by a set of material practices, signs, figures, superstitions, images and fictions that, because they are available to individuals' imagination and intelligence and actually experienced, form what might be called 'languages of life'" (Mbembe, 2001). A circumstantial and innovative attention to power potentially provides us with tools to sustain understandings of the ways in which the "action of knowledge" influence and act on its "field of operation"

(Race, 2001). This type of enquiry will allow us to discard the view that knowledge and its productions are neutral, rational, and proceeds through calculative processes. Rather, "knowledge and its mechanisms are capable of generating a set of affective consequences. In fact they are capable of producing subjects" (Race, 2001). This "subject creation" might not correlate to "normal" processes of citizenship formation but are becoming increasingly "normal" in light of increasing states of exception and crises that are marking our contemporary global situation.

Judith Butler (1990), in a similar vein, indicates that "truth effects" are produced through a process of "reiterative repetition." In the case of HIV and AIDS, ordinary people as well as academics hear, see, feel, and produce the same concepts, categorizations, and typologies associated with our specific HIV and AIDS "zeitgeist" that circulate in research, in the popular media, therefore in mainstream discourses that reign supreme at a specific point in time and whereby HIV and AIDS is fetishized according to these dominant views.

The hypocrisies of HIV research

"People with HIV/AIDS are a vulnerable group that should be protected from researchers" Ambrose Rachier at the 12th World AIDS Conference during the session titled: "Bridging Session: Ethics & Science" in July 1998.

(in Kopp, 2002)

It was shown in the previous section the extent to which knowledge formation, and therefore affiliated representations, have been largely contingent upon specific historical and social contexts and accepted global moral economies which allow the circulation and enforcement of truth claims. These are now increasingly critiqued although critique thereof does not seem to influence the manner in which certain "at risk" groups are still framed and acted on. One such example is the manner in which HIV experts initially made very significant and far-reaching knowledge claims about the possibilities of ART, as well as about potential drug resistance in Africa, and this without recourse to strong empirical research on this sensitive topic. Given the widespread biomedicalized normalization and the maturation of the availability of ART, it is inevitable that drug resistance will also be increasing. However, the battle is still being fought to resist dominant discourses that concentrate mainly on individual failures to drug adherence, spilling over into those reasons most widely cited to make sense of treatment failure. Issues of ART adherence (like with TB treatment adherence or any other form of sustained and disciplined observance) is actually much more dependent on issues of continued (at times, more expensive) medical access (second- and third-line therapy regimens) and on structural explanations. Those becoming resistant to ART often do not have recourse to taken-for-granted resources, such as time, transport money, or social capital. These behaviors which are generally and simplistically ascribed to recalcitrant individual defaulting only become truly comprehensible through narratives that appeal and convince when told through real-life stories of those often confined to statistical renditions of "successes and failures" (Farmer, 1999; Biehl & Petryna, 2013). Other forms of triage, apart from flagrant denial of treatment to poor people, are also responsible for forms of resistance that might soon become much more of a reality, especially (and non-surprisingly) in resource-constrained settings. These issues of triage are less linked to behavior and much more to structural understandings of the manner in which drug prices are decided on, the availability and affordability of the most effective medicines (for example dolutegravir as the most effective first-line treatment, and access to third-line regimens), and the manner in which Intellectual Property is legislated, enforced, and allowed to dictate the manner in which drugs are developed and dispersed.[2] These divergent views of simplified notions, such as "drug resistance" and "treatment non-adherence," shed light as to the complexities of issues of HIV and treatment as they currently unfold at the coalface. It is, therefore, imperative to understand how these wider institutional and social spin-offs of the HIV and AIDS world conform to the "social realities imposed by global regulartory organizations" (Hunt, 1997). We too often stop with critical engagements once success stories are heralded of certain (aimed for) outcomes that today might seem to come closer to the 90:90:90 targets set by the UNAIDS in 2015. These success stories are often confined to places of easy access and where the researched "do not talk back" (Smith, 2012). It has been indicated that AIDS researchers and others who work in certain settings, especially in Africa

> too often content themselves with success stories, produced in countries where expatriates feel welcome and can easily get around and out again, and where functioning medical systems provide amenable working conditions. Yet AIDS research capitals keep shifting in relation to stability, access, and crises.
>
> (Hunt, 1997)

Responding to issues of access and crises, PEPFAR represented the "largest ever international public health program" (Rottenburg, 2009) and boasted the largest spending any particular government has ever contributed toward a single disease internationally. The bulk of PEPFAR funding is directed toward funding a variety of HIV and AIDS interventions in Africa, and therefore, this program has also introduced an era of unparalleled commitment in African health by the American state and its collaborating institutions. It is also noteworthy that PEPFAR money travels not only through the State Department and government agencies (the US Agency for International Development [USAID] and Centers for Disease Control and Prevention [CDC]) but also through both public and private US universities. According to Crane (2013), in 2007, the top three of the ten PEPFAR grant beneficiaries were, in fact, American universities engaged in HIV treatment and prevention services, as well as vaccine research in 13 countries, 12 of which were located within sub-Saharan Africa. She continues to track the involvement of Northern American institution in an era of AIDS in Africa by stating that the global health programs of the USA and Canadian universities tripled between the years 2006 and 2011 which is truly indicative of the "enthusiasm for global health within the North American academy" (Doughton, 2011, in Crane, 2013).

In light of this proliferation of research activities and the influx of academics from the global North into the environment of the global South, Nancy Rose Hunt's forewarnings as early on as in 1997 now ring more true than ever. She specified that it is now more important than ever to understand where "innovative, ethical, and thoughtful work" is being done on HIV and AIDS and which discourses to regard with suspicion. The informed knowledge of who is doing what and the manner in which these endeavors address the most relevant ethical considerations of the moment also stretches into the actual field in which academics continue to perform their research activities. Research participants or people living with HIV and AIDS (PLWHAs) are becoming increasingly disillusioned and skeptical about the ease with which international and local researchers move into and out of communities of people and leave as abruptly with their "findings" that are subsequently neatly exposed and reported at the manifold conferences that report about these issues and those represented. In fact, at the 7th South African AIDS Conference in June 2015 in Durban, the national secretary of National Association of People Living With HIV/AIDS (NAPWA) voiced his dissatisfaction with the manner in which the Human Science Research Council (HSRC) "used" the organization, NAPWA in order to customize the Stigma Index Questionnaire for this authoritative study that took place for the first time in South Africa, the findings of which were presented at this conference. NAPWA was the proverbial "participant," the HSRC filling the role of the stereotypical "researcher." Does this increasingly prevalent disillusionment mean an end to HIV-related fieldwork? Have we reached a point of "saturation," both as researchers and as communities? Are we now simply flogging the proverbial dead horse because there is some money left in partially spent research projects or because of the fact that HIV happens to be so many academics' niche area of research? Are the studies that we perform done truly to benefit communities or to merely lead to conjuring up academic argumentations, that at times become increasingly removed from the original source. Communities that are willing to partake in these studies often do so because participation in trials or other research studies might harbor potential advantages that are normally not available to these individuals, the apogée being to participate in a drug trial where care is, under normal circumstances, significantly worse or nonexistent. This might lead to the "bio-availability" of bodies, more so poor women's bodies (as they tend to enroll more often in health-related research studies), "for the exploitation in an era of global capitalism" (Cohen, 2005). Africa continues to be, in too many ways, simply the field site where research respondents and participants are much more freely and easily available, the "raw material" of data to be produced and packaged as the feats of researchers who are geographically, emotionally, and intellectually removed from the continuing everyday realities of the participants' plight. And this might even be the case of so-called "local" researchers who might be geographically close to study participants, but geographic location is where this proximity ends and intersectional privilege starts.

Outcome expediency is also inscribed into the various endeavors enacted by those operating in the field of HIV. One example thereof was indicated in Nguyen's (2010) findings of early initiatives, under the auspices of UNAIDS to provide highly active ART to some eligible candidates in the Ivory Coast when this treatment first became available in Africa more widely. Only two, instead of three, drugs were subsidized during this initiative. Local authorities still continued with the roll-out of this insufficient treatment regime (two, instead of three, lines of treatment), knowing very well what the consequences of such an action would be. He found that this initiative "was more about showing that something was being done for political ends both domestically and internationally than about achieving meaningful public health results" (Nguyen, 2010). Even then, knowledge as to the effects of this exercise was available as these two drugs would only be partially effective at suppressing the virus and would, therefore, give the virus time to become resistant to this inadequate drug regimen. The reason that was provided to Nguyen for this practice was that it allowed the authorities to reach more patients that could benefit from ARTs (Nguyen, 2010). In so many ways, Uganda's HIV and AIDS narrative has also been flaunted as "a success story" that could be transplanted to the rest of "Africa" in an attempt to curb the onslaught of HIV and AIDS in sub-Saharan Africa and elsewhere where HIV prevalence was high. The "Ugandan Experience" was the prototype prioritized by the UNAIDS despite evidence from social scientists that started pointing to differing interpretations (Pigg, 2013).

Outcome expediency, or rather political expediency, is prominent in the current climate of global health with an increased focus on technical approaches to remedy health-related issues. This can be seen by what has been termed the "private turn" in global health governance as state systems and even traditional international bodies, such as the World Health Organization (WHO) are increasingly marginalized to respond to disease manifestation. Influential organizations, such as the Gates Foundations, are focused on developing top-down interventions (Rushton & Williams, 2011), valuing quantifiable outcomes, and sidelining basic public health which, contrary to a technological, top-down approach, rather encapsulates responses to disease that

> address the health needs of a population or the collective health status of the people rather than focusing primarily on individual case management. This approach aims to ensure the widest possible access to high quality services at the population level, based on simplified and

standardized approaches, and to strike a balance between implementing the best-proven standard of care and what is feasible on a large scale in resource-limited settings. For HIV, key elements of a public health approach include simplified drug formularies; large-scale use of fixed-dose combinations for first-line treatment for adults, adolescents and children; care and drugs provided free at the point of service delivery; decentralization and integration of services, including task shifting; and simplified approaches to clinical monitoring.

(WHO, 2015b)

The diminishing role of a quintessential public health, horizontal approach to respond to diseases and epidemics is driving global health policy more generally toward technical interventions where problem, cause, and effect can be quantified, costed, and compared with others. This is evident in the growing influence of "audit cultures" within healthcare administration as well as the development of institution in the USA such as the Institute for Health Metrics and Evaluation (IHME), a new initiative based at the University of Washington which is largely funded by the Bill and Melinda Gates Foundation (Crane, 2013). The vision of the IHME is vested in health improvement through applying scientific rationalism. Managerialist jargon is increasingly infiltrating the HIV and AIDS domain where proposals for performance-based incentives (PBIs) for the prevention of HIV transmission are indicative the manner in which this "intensified therapeutic neoliberalism – where a rational economic calculus is brought to bear on all aspects of life pertaining to HIV and AIDS – might look like at the level of managerial techniques and modes of subjectification" (Ingram, 2013). Over (2010) explains that PBI's main purpose is to "adjust individual agents' incentives to better align with the interests of the community and the country." This economistic and managerialist discourse continues to dictate that PBI's would mean that "on the demand side, they should heighten the interest of individual clients. On the supply side, they should motivate service providers to try harder" (Ingram, 2013).

This idea is increasingly gaining currency among donors globally in order to quantify, predict, and prove intervention outcomes. Efficiency is the new donor mantra, resonating with broader issues of neoliberalism and market fundamentalism that increasingly include the calculation of scarcity and of retrenchment. All of these shifts in donor sentiments and actions have tremendous repercussions for the manner in which HIV and AIDS initiatives will attract and retain donor support in contemporary times.

The focus of intervening into the lives of those far from the global North is also in stark contrast to issues that happen closer to home. The fervor with which organizations scrambled to share in the pickings of the global AIDS pie (especially by intervening in the global South) is ironic given that the African American community in the USA is one of the groups that is disproportionately affected by HIV infection within the USA. Those lobbying for HIV interventions in the USA are rightfully comparing their HIV rates in the USA to those in Africa. In 2008, a report indicated that "the number of people living with HIV in Black America exceed the HIV populations in 7 of the 15 focus countries of the U.S. government's PEPFAR initiative" (Wilson et al., 2008). The rationality of some initial and even some contemporary interventions in the emergence of an exceptional epidemic, such as HIV, is definitely not always evident, as can be explained by many dubious practices.

The place of the "lesser" scientists

The growth and importance of the social sciences was instrumental to the initial reliance on technical development and its various promises to lend assistance to the "developing world" (Packard, 2016). The social sciences provided the necessary theoretical foundations that were needed to rationalize and justify the variety of efforts by European countries and North America aimed at transforming the "developing world through technical assistance." As these technical progressions developed over the years, studying the actual "culture of development" was, however, less appreciated by this "technical-assistance community" that social sciences helped to create in the first place (Packard, 2016).

The normalization and increased focus on biomedicalization processes of the HIV epidemic have plunged social and cultural sciences into a variety of crises of legitimacy as to these disciplines' continued relevance within this contemporary therapeutic scenario. This epidemic of "signification" (Treichler, 1999) was initially coined as such, given the terrain of uncertainty that AIDS emphasized on so many levels. It being an epidemic of signification simply meant that there were few clear referents to deal with the manner in which the disease took root in such diverse contexts and with such multiple ramifications. Thus, the notion of its signification thus opened various possibilities of interpretation and of sense-making, in order to prevent and to resist finality and closure of something as seemingly complex as a disease, but in actual fact much more intelligible as an illness. Framing an epidemic as such allows social and cultural scientists with a productive environment in which to be attuned to larger processes of meaning production and of representation. However, with normalization comes processes of increased focus on problems rather narrowly defined in order to enhance and entrench the current technical and technological "quick-fix" solutions mostly enshrined in a growing emphasis on "evidence-based" research that is mustered in order to cement this growing ubiquity of biomedical normalization. These processes then are increasingly focused on directing interventions and to a lesser extent is the focus (or rather, the funding) directed to the interventions that actually work. In the past and continuing today, social and cultural sciences' theories added a lot in terms of describing the dynamics of the HIV epidemic, but it too rarely resulted in informing specific responses to the epidemic

(Mykhalovskiy & Rosengarten, 2009). The "mania for measurement" (Posel, 2000), mostly through the use of randomized control trials, have become the ultimate gold standard with which knowledge is adjudicated, legitimized, and acted on.

Social and cultural sciences, moreover social and cultural sciences from non-hegemonic intellectual geographies (i.e. the global South) are often underrepresented in global academic discourses despite the fact that it is within these areas where epidemics wreck the most havoc. Research is, therefore, also increasingly critical of the geographical location where specific interpretations are generated. This phenomenon is indicative of the unequal conceptual generative force that was unleashed in the AIDS aftermath, yet another derivative of the AIDS industry. In 2013, an astounding 52% of research on HIV and AIDS was produced in the USA and the UK only (identified in the Web of Science Core Collection; Collyer, 2015 in Hodes & Morrell, 2018) despite the greatest majority of HIV-infected people not living in these geographical locations. Scholars and activists from the global South have often argued that knowledge production, even when it focuses on issues pertaining to the lives of people in the South, including HIV and AIDS, generally tends to be dominated by scholars and institutions from the academic "global North" (especially those from Europe and North America; see Adams et al., 2010). Research elsewhere has also noted this inequality in knowledge generation and dissemination. For example, a study conducted by a Chilean nongovernmental organization (NGO; Fallabela et al., 2009) found that scholars from the South tend to be sidelined from knowledge production and dissemination in key platforms, including academic journals. Reasons for this include language barriers (with English being the dominant language of research and publication), the complex nature of the academic discourses needed to generate and communicate knowledge, and the general marginalization of knowledge produced by local southern communities (Fallabela et al., 2009). This state of affairs potentially harbors the effect of furthering the global asymmetries not only of disease manifestation but also in the labor of knowledge production. The view from the so-called South[3] might in the process be severely eschewed, despite the global emphasis that is increasingly calling for processes of decolonization (Connell et al., 2018). However, to somehow counter this status quo, South African authors Rebecca Hodes and Robert Morrell (2018) indicate that the ten most cited social sciences papers produced by South Africans have, contrary to expectations, actually introduced a "research agenda and challenged core conceptualizations of HIV epidemiology" (Hodes & Morrell, 2018). These authors contend that inasmuch as "Southern" social scientists work with concepts generated in the "North," this endeavor is not uncritical or unidirectional but equally include notions of reciprocity and relationality (Hodes & Morrell, 2018). It will be revealing to study the manner in which research produced elsewhere in the global South (especially from other African countries) similarly influence the wider academic discourses produced about AIDS and its derivatives.

In light of a recent call by UNAIDS (2014b, 2016) to find "new biosocial" responses to complement the biomedical treatment of HIV is rather surprising if not patently ludicrous. This call is expressed in the midst of heaps of information where caution for detail and context of the minutiae of unfolding realities – ever so complex, transforming, reconfiguring, and mutable – can simply be replaced by a process or an initiative where some "new" findings potentially conceal the "new biosocial" response to this hybrid state of being. This is evident in the manner in which "social scientists" or other stakeholders are trying to discover the holy grail of seemingly elusive biosocial explanations and responses. A recent article (Burman, 2018), for example, configures "a novel agenda," titled "The Taming Wicked Problems Framework," presenting a "nascent biosocial candidate to reinforce the biomedical strategy" of the UNAIDS 90:90:90 goal-setting with the ultimate aim of ending AIDS by 2030. This framework aims to realign management techniques in order to respond to the nonlinear and complex nature that always associates intervention actions, moreover those associated with HIV and AIDS. Heeding this type of call is baffling seeing that it takes place in a vacuum, ignoring years of evidence that has developed to explicate the (complex) reasons behind the specific manifestations of HIV infection and its persistence in the first place, and the manifold reasons (complex and nonlinear) that are behind failures, unintended (even perverse) outcomes, or short-term successes of interventions. Is this perhaps indicative of the low regard that social sciences with complex, nuanced renditions of the epidemic have had to endure in the past and in times to come? Provided that resources are becoming increasingly limited, it goes without saying that these are the intellectual spaces that will feel the plateauing of HIV and AIDS research most acutely. These intellectual disciplines will have to adapt to the type of evidence-based, managerialist, and cost-effective dictates that are increasingly characterizing HIV and AIDS in the global health context. Peter Piot, the once director of UNAIDS indicated as much when he emphasized the increasing role that social scientists could play to contribute in a very *operational way* to the interventions that those with decision-making power decide on (Piot, 2008).

Those engaged with social sciences and humanities research felt the urgent need to create their own organization to deal with the structural and the psychological dimensions of this devastating and complex phenomenon that is HIV and AIDS. As one of the organization's founding members, Dr Judy Auerbach explained it, the Association for Social Sciences and Humanities in HIV (ASSHH – pronounced *"ash"*) came into existence because of feelings of exclusion and isolation and being ignored by the mainstream (i.e. biomedical) HIV and AIDS world of research, funding, policy, and decision making. However, the association's future is precarious, as was evident during the 2015 conference in Stellenbosch, South Africa. Antagonisms between important stakeholders that led to divisions about future funding options meant that the organization is teetering to maintain its short-lived presence, despite a conference having been hosted at the Amsterdam Institute for Global

Health & Development (but not under the banner of ASSHH). Their website also does not seem to be in existence any longer. This unfortunate turn of events is perhaps pointing to the de-legitimized role that social sciences and humanities still occupy in the larger HIV and AIDS landscape, moreover if the reason behind ASSHH's demise is rooted at the level of non-reconcilable differences between various stakeholders.

Provided that the field of HIV and AIDS is ever-evolving with levels of complexity that are far from abating, there will always be the intense need to respond to Paula Treichler's (1999) question: "How do ordinary people make sense of a novel cultural phenomenon that is complicated and unpredictable" (such as HIV and AIDS)? As discussed in previous chapters, a default approach involves framing the new (or evolving) phenomenon within familiar narratives. This can also involve a "looking back and going back to our roots" approach, a nostalgia for the past which seeks to restore what was lost (Boym, 2001) as people grapple with the new and often daunting phenomena. It might also manifest in an increasingly belligerent attitude among those who are still pursuing research in this field, but within disciplines that are increasingly de-legitimized and disregarded by means of cutting funds but also by seeking so-called "new" biosocial responses to support the processes of medicalization and normalization.

The way forward

Our sole legitimacy to speak and our sole claim to be listened to depend on our capacity to contest untested assumptions, the most insidious being that on which we found our moral certainties.

(Fassin, 2012b)

From an interpretivist stance, we understand that the social world is ultimately a world that we create. By studying this social world, we are in a constant process of re-creating it. This re-creation is important as it can lead to transformation which again needs to fit into the circularity of enquiry in order to gauge the results, intended or not, of transformations. It is for this reason and to learn from past experiences that academic accounts are increasingly focused on reflecting on the contentious and interpretative nature of "successes" and "failures" in HIV and AIDS research practices (Kingori & Sariola, 2015).

Social enquiries into the now prevalent biomedical interventions can roughly be categorized into two distinct approaches, both sorely needed for responsive future interventions but also needed to disallow the easy approach of venturing into the dangerous and gaping Luddite trap. First, there is the body of literature that (rightly) sings the praise of ART: its life-giving abilities, rendering HIV into a chronic condition and no longer a death sentence, empowering those who ingest it, as well as those who benefit from it indirectly (be it the labor market, families, communities, etc.), and its capabilities to give rise to new demands in relation to claims to citizenship, even to "thin citizenship." But second, there is also a growing (and needed) literature that could be deemed "critical literature" that speaks of experiences from the field, where treatment might be denied or where incorrect procedures might give rise to problems with treatment. Being "critical" of the production of scientific knowledge does not (necessarily) mean being dismissive of foundational epistemological claims of contemporary science. Rather, as indicated by Geffen and Gonsalves (2008), it implies framing the complex processes that are associated with the production and application of knowledge as decision making that is always both technical and political. Although this critical enquiry of HIV science has been in existence for a number of years, these are the kinds of questions that are becoming increasingly difficult to ask in times of normalization and biomedicalization and accompanying HIV scale-up. These processes are rather viewed as problematic sets of "technical problems." Within this technical complexities that we are witnessing today, activists could then at times be "overplaying unproved but sensational misdeeds" (as we explained in Chapter 4) and thereby obscure the more serious ones. This "scattershot" approach to the ethics around HIV and AIDS "draws attention away from a critical and increasingly complicated issue that AIDS has pushed to the fore ..." (Cohen, 2006). Being able to discern between those ethical aspects that are deemed "rational" and worth pursuing in this period of normalization is, therefore, becoming progressively more intricate. The exact and most relevant future not only of biomedical scientific progress but also ethically sound and relevant social scientific enquiry needs to be responsive to this new era of heightened demands of accountability and scrutiny. The current period of normalizing HIV and its treatment and the sustained ability to guarantee effective and long-term interventions at scale will not automatically happen, as is often deemed by technocrats and politicians whose focus is on scientific and political expediency. Enquiries into the complications of these interventions are, in today's era of normalization, often seen as exaggerated or even monotonous and passé with its continued focus on those structural and seemingly reified arrangements that are almost always at the root of epidemics' spread and responses. With biomedical progress and ever-transforming abilities rooted in improved molecular science, clinical innovations lead to more effective treatments, although this happens largely by way of stratification. These innovations inspire optimisms for improved and more targeted treatment options. However, this progress also provokes major dilemmas around treatment availability, equity of treatment access, and the social formations of care, thus rearticulating forms of biological and social stratification, with important implications for the manner in which lives are deemed valuable enough to save or to improve the experience of those infected with HIV.

Nguyen (2004) has indicated that claims gravitating around HIV and AIDS have been more successful to unleash international attention than claims that were founded simply on poverty and its accompanying plights that affect so many people on this planet. With the end of AIDS exceptionality, global

AIDS activism finds itself lost in the quagmire of issues that have become largely banal and diffuse. Activism has been an exemplary outflow of AIDS exceptionalism, and its continued actions perhaps the only way in which urgency and attention to HIV as well as to its manifold ramifications might be sustained. Chris Colvin (2014) suggests some actions as to the manner in which activism could be taken into what he calls "third wave" advocacy. This third wave is associated with those complications characteristic of a generalized epidemic and the widespread availability of ART: activism beyond the era of emergency and urgency.

He first suggests to "engage more fully with the mundane as a political problem and terrain" (Colvin, 2014). Here he emphasizes the importance of activist-academic links to render this engagement with the quotidian feasible and capable of generating much-needed empirical evidence. In South Africa, the Treatment Action Campaign (TAC) has taken to task this engagement with the everyday by reporting on these seemingly banal issues that could have disastrous consequences for those affected by it. Their attention to drug stock-outs and the day-to-day operational aspects of ART are cases in point. So too is attention to "mundane tasks of health financing, long-term maintenance of behaviour change, supply-chain management and careful realignment of primary health care services" (Colvin, 2014). The TAC's compilation of the Health Report where ordinary people's experiences of the Free State public healthcare system was highlighted, accentuates some truly incriminating detail of "the everyday" that is, in fact, in direct opposition to people's respect, dignity, and human rights. Mundane, therefore, does not mean unimportant although there might not necessarily be "straightforward or dramatic solutions" (Colvin, 2014). These micro-issues are ultimately what add up to culminate into people's experiences of the much-vaunted macro-processes of biomedicalization and widespread sentiments of normalization.

Second, Colvin (2014) states the important issue of democratizing evidence, "both in terms of access and production." The history of AIDS exceptionalism has been shown to have democratized evidence in unprecedented ways, breaking the historical distinction that was (and still is) drawn between "expert" and "lay" health knowledge. In the initial years of the HIV epidemic, it was shown how individuals gained increasing knowledge and expertise of highly technical biomedical information that directly affected their own health concerns (Petryna, 2002; Rose, 2007; Nguyen, 2010; Young, 2015). However, the generative force of the epidemic that led to the early years of vibrant activism also waned after ART became widely available.

With the burgeoning emergence of a variety of participatory politics that HIV and AIDS ushered in (through activism and through the establishment and concretization of community healthcare), some scholars in the South African context tend

to overstate the organizational strengths of embryonic forms of community-based organization and social movements. As is always the case, history and developments expose this form of "romanticism" when these organizations collapse and when they face deep divisions based on internal strategic and tactical differences.

(Runciman, 2015)

Although internal conflicts were always present within the South African HIV and AIDS domain (as was witnessed with the early acrimony between the TAC and NAPWA), processes of normalization and biomedicalization also lead to largely depoliticizing HIV and AIDS, thereby rendering its science less accountable to those whose lives are directly influenced by it. For example, it is telling that in the TAC's 2017 Resolution Document, resolution 36.1 indicated "funding permitting, TAC will revive our Treatment Literacy presence in health facilities with Provincial Treatment Literacy people and branch organizers providing Treatment Literacy education in health facilities and communities." The treatment literacy used to be a flagship advocacy initiative that largely marked the successful years of activism not only globally but also in South Africa. In order to democratize evidence, this treatment literacy of the biomedical aspects of HIV kept ordinary lay people abreast of the manners in which treatment is evolving.

Also, for the social sciences, new methodologies and reflections on the manner in which knowledge is generated and representations crafted should become mainstream in taking HIV and AIDS research forward. Ethical ways of doing research – that does not merely comply with those mechanistic ethical requirements too often ascribed to by Ethics Review Boards (following the biomedical model and tick-box procedures) – should be debated, developed, and embraced. Issues such as "non-mastery" (Lather, 2002), "situatedness," "partiality" (Jungar & Oinas, 2011), and going back to initial concept formation, propensities, and ideas (as was done by Jonny Steinberg, 2016) are now more needed than ever in order for social scientific research to remain relevant and ethically accountable in taking HIV and AIDS research to the next level. Involving those whose lives are most affected will also democratize research participation and remedy asymmetries that normally mark the conventional manner in which research is configured (Africa being the extractivist research site where those with more access to a variety of capital benefit from generating their ideas, concepts, or medical breakthroughs). Initiatives such as the 2000 Nairobi Declaration (an African Appeal for an AIDS Vaccine), where African countries were to become more involved in vaccine trials, need to be supported and developed. This is echoed by a more recent initiative called the Globally Relevant AIDS Vaccine Europe-Africa Trials Partnership (GREAT), initiated by the International AIDS Vaccine Initiative (IAVI) to evaluate a promising vaccine known as tHIVconsvX. This vaccine is aimed at targeting the challenging issue of HIV mutations and is indicative of a wider collaboration between the global South and the global North (IAVI, 2017).

In light of biomedical cooperation and progress, Colvin's (2014) third and last recommendation is critical in that it cautions that in order to take activism into an age of normalization, it will have to "move beyond some of the conventional kinds of 'data-driven advocacy'" and "to promote the production and deployment of new forms of evidence that are 'critical' in perspective and independent of existing institutional and hegemonic modes of knowledge production." This recommendation is especially prescient in light of the narrowing-down of evidence-based interventions that social scientists are often co-opted into in order to adjudicate successes and failures. This does not easily allow for evidence to stand apart from politics, as the "answers" are in the data. Nathan Geffen and Gregg Gonsalves (2008) argue that activists need "clear" scientific evidence and internationally recognized guidelines in order to bring pressure on governments to provide services to its citizens. But if activists are only to rely on state-sanctioned forms of "knowledge [created] for governing healthcare" (Mykhalovskiy & Rosengarten, 2009) such as "evidence-based norms and standards," activists may find themselves increasingly co-opted in both a discourse and a practice of evidence that reproduce some of the worst elements of the status quo.

Research that is relevant and reflective and steeped in forms of activism is one productive and potentially rewarding way to broach the future of HIV enquiry and concomitant actions such as intervention and policy formulations. The pitfalls are widely strewn given the collateral damage inherent in processes of normalization, as was indicated in the preceding chapters. Taking activism seriously as a way to continue with relevant HIV and AIDS research is because of the fact that activism has, in the words of Jungar and Oinas (2011),

> both implicitly and explicitly destabilized the cherished images and formulae we use to identify agency, power and resistance. Despite the "best intentions" of their producers, these images and formulae easily reinforce the dualisms, silences and hierarchies that have historically elevated certain bodies' normalcy and power, and entrenched the silence, invisibility and inferiority of others. The activist approach to the HIV epidemic, embodiment and the social order challenges existing discourses in ways that oblige us to revisit some of our most fundamental assumptions about embodied experiences.

Activism, combined with research, is needed to come up with examples of "pragmatic solidarity," in the words of Paul Farmer (2000) whose groundbreaking intellectual perspectives are couched in lengthy field experiences in places and of conditions largely neglected in the global moral economy as it is currently configured. Activism, combining science with advocacy by detailing lived experiences and structural constraints, and culminating into informed knowledge gain as well as knowledge generation, is what an ideal future looks like in the domain of ethical HIV and AIDS research. HIV and AIDS activism has given rise to the emergence of a powerful sense of rights, not only to treatment but also a sense of right to life and of responsibilities to others, as indicated by Nguyen (2010). Nguyen's (2010) depiction of this unique "therapeutic citizenship" differs from other forms of "biological citizenship" as authoritatively described by Petryna (2002) and Rose and Novas (2004). This is largely because Nguyen's development of "therapeutic citizenship" is based on a "thin citizenship" where the focus is only on one disease and the accompanying interests that directly influence the level of commitment to and legitimacy of this epidemic. The manifestation of this "therapeutic citizenship" in places where other forms of citizenship are at times in short supply to those infected and affected by the epidemic is what renders the normalization thereof all the more worrisome. As Nguyen (2010) indicates,

> since it is active in a setting where the disease may be the only way to get any of the material security one usually associates with citizenship, it takes on a particular poignancy.

Conclusion

Whereas some social scientific endeavors of the past are (easily) criticized today for being too eagerly co-opted into the dominant status quo of their time and of being the handmaiden of colonialism in many instances, this critique is more complicated in our contemporary times given the manner in which social scientific contributions to diseases are, in turn, becoming increasingly complicit with neoliberal dictates and dependent on outcome expediency. Ethical imperatives of doing relevant research are often translated into doing something concrete and applied, with the eye on empirical evidence of outcomes and results. Stacey Leigh Pigg (2013) invites us to "pause in the eddies created by the forward momentum of global health activity" as a potential way of "doing" research. This reiterates the ethical predicament, so well described by Didier Fassin (2012b), where he captures the continued contradiction faced by those studying the social side of disease, where we find ourselves "between the ethical affirmation of the superior value of life and the empirical acknowledgement of the unequal worth of lives" and where it becomes all the more important to negotiate this "fine line between scientific detachment and moral involvement" to make a "modest but crucial contribution to society – and in the present case – to global health." In doing this, social scientists add the element of critical thinking in order to understand and not only to denounce the injustices of the current configuration of global health and its widespread ramifications (Fassin, 2012b). Social scientists' closeness in the field often allows a look at "institutional dynamics that would predict the imperviousness in development institutions" and allows us to look at the present with the attention, called "imponderabilia,"[4] that Malinowski argued, was necessary. This would allow the critical dispensation which is now urgently needed, in order to focus on the "present" instead of on a view of "social engineering of a particular future" (Pigg, 2013). The importance of contextually rich, non-static, and highly contingent factors, interweaving especially in contexts of precariousness, should also continually juxtapose – as has been evident in the South African HIV domain – the intricate interplay of "marginality in relation to HIV infection and transmission, [and] how to account for the determinism of structural legacies, while avowing the dynamism of social change" where the medical and the social are co-constituted and co-produced; dialectical rather than dichotomized (Hodes & Morrell, 2018).

Notes

1 These words were uttered by the then deputy president of South Africa (currently president), Cyril Ramaphosa, during a plenary speech at the 2015 South African AIDS Conference in Durban. He spoke in his capacity as president of the South African National Council on HIV and AIDS (SANAC).

2 In the 2017 TAC resolutions, Resolution 47 makes mention of the situation that is "morally unacceptable that many medicines are unavailable or unaffordable" within South Africa. The TAC, therefore, vouches to advance activism that "will bring about a more rational and humane policy and legal framework to guide how society pays for existing medicines and for the research and development of new medicines." The campaign titled "Fix the Patent Laws" that has been running for some time now, is indicative of this strategic move (TAC, 2018).

3 Southern theory is not necessarily confined to a specific geographical location (according to Dados & Connell, 2012, in Hodes & Morrell, 2018) but rather to "their critical engagement with how knowledge is produced along global axes of affluence, prestige and power."

4 Pigg (2013) indicates what Malinowski implied, by "imponderabilia." This is a process of capturing, through ethnographic investigation, the "mood, tone, sensory experience, and the mundane" which has the potential to lead to "a transformative insight into others' points of view," and in this process, "others' experience becomes possible."

Conclusion

The future of HIV and AIDS in terms of successfully managing this social epidemic is in peril. This book is an account which traces the configuration of AIDS as an exceptional disease. This was done by merely pointing to some arbitrary occurrences – occurrences among many other – to make this argument. From a mere biomedical perspective, the immense successes that have marked HIV and AIDS treatments have to be aligned in such a way to translate HIV care and prevention that benefit individuals into population-wide advantages. However, as we saw in Chapter 2, fiscal constraints and global austerity create an environment that challenges a clear-cut biomedical victory over the epidemic. In addition to simple treatment and its potential successful outcomes, HIV is also a problem to treat in populations that are hard to reach – often these are the groups most in need of HIV care. To control the HIV epidemic will remain elusive if the interruption of infection does not occur within high-incidence settings. In addition, those individuals who have been reached need to be retained in care in order to pursue successful treatment regimens with the ultimate aim to lead to sustainable viral suppression levels. The challenges are many, but AIDS exceptionalism and its concomitant assemblages have given rise to a solid biomedical establishment to grapple with these issues. This establishment, part of the AIDS industry, still holds sway as they are the champions of biomedicalization and its accompanying promises. There is still tremendous energy and vitality in biomedical AIDS work, as is evident by the amount of literature that tracks biomedical progress as well as the amount of research that is being done and money that is being invested into HIV and AIDS. It would also be unfair to say that the South African biomedical AIDS establishment gleans over social issues of the disease. Like elsewhere in the globe, there has been tremendous cooperation and knowledge exchange between scientists and activists, and this feature continues to mark the South African HIV and AIDS landscape. Biomedicalization has largely brought about the positive aspects of normalization inasmuch as HIV and AIDS is less stigmatized and more manageable to those who are securely on treatment.

However, no establishment is immune to severe budget cuts nor to curtailing directives that do not allow measures of freedom to imagine future research practices and interventions. The global donor establishment, in line with global health's increased focus on vertical, cost-effective, and evidence-based interventions, increasingly functions within these stifling parameters. Global health should continue to pursue its cosmopolitan nature (Pogge, 2002) and thereby to extend the narrow focus of justice beyond the nation-state. In fact, this cosmopolitanism of rights has been the one feature of HIV and AIDS that rendered it exceptional soon after its emergence. This was witnessed by the immense cooperation and exchanges between activists around the globe. Sustaining this activism, albeit with a focus that "breaks out of the disease constituency model" (Epstein in Mykhalovskiy & Rosengarten, 2009), is the only maintainable future to normalized AIDS. Expanding cosmopolitan rights to other instances of social injustices is what makes this potential future of activism and advocacy ethically appealing. The search for viable and sustainable activism is also needed more than ever in a world where right-wing libertarianism with narrow individualistic approaches to human rights and justice as well as "cost-effective utilitarianism" (Mbali, 2013) are defining the contours of social justice more generally. In increased instances of "exceptionalizing" issues in order to create Naomi Klein's "democracy-free zones," it is only through the work of informed, energetic, and sustained activism that these issues could be made known to the world.

In addition, human rights are increasingly under threat as was presciently indicated by Hannah Arendt in her trenchant critique of this concept (Arendt, 1968). She indicated that for humans to have rights, we need to be *more than merely human*, we need to have the "right to have rights." We can lay claim to our rights only if we belong to some form of political community. Activism is one form of citizenship claiming, together with other forms of "self-fashioning" to enhance forms of belonging and identity. This reading of Arendt obviously makes a lot of sense in our contemporary times where millions of people are displaced because of war, conflict, persecution, or natural disasters. However, in the world of epidemics and our vulnerability to it, it has been shown throughout this book (and by an array of excellent academic accounts) that HIV and notions of citizenship are intricately enmeshed, as was shown in both chapters on Community Health Workers and on AIDS activism. AIDS exceptionality somehow paved the way for the creation of new forms of citizenship and to the shaping of a unique approach to the exercise of human rights within South Africa. This process is not perfect and flawless, but it nonetheless opened up interesting and promising spaces of expression that will persist for a long time to come, given the reconfiguration, especially in South Africa, of activism beyond HIV and beyond exceptionality, but still critically relevant to this country and also to the world, to imagine a better future for all global citizens.

Bibliography

Abdool Karim, S. & Abdool Karim, Q., 2016. Durban: From AIDS 2000 to AIDS 2016. In: Treatment Action Campaign & Section 27. *AIDS Durban 2000–2016*. Johannesburg: Treatment Action Campaign & Section 27, pp. 19–21.

Adams, J., King, C. & Hook, D., 2010. Global Research Report: Africa. *Eldis* [Online] Available at: www.eldis.org/document/A51711. [Accessed 10 May 2018].

Agamben, G., 1998. *Homo Sacer: Sovereign Power and Bare Life*. Stanford: Stanford University Press.

Ahmad, H., 2013. The Treatment Action Campaign and the Three Dimensions of Lawyering: Reflections from the Rainbow Nation. *Journal of Social Aspects of HIV/AIDS*, 10(1), pp. 17–24.

Appadurai, A., 2001. Deep Democracy: Urban Governmentality and the Horizon of Politics. *Environment & Urbanization*, 13, pp. 23–44.

Arendt, H., 1968. *The Origins of Totalitarianism* (new edition). San Diego: Harvest.

Avert, 2019. *Funding for HIV and AIDS*. [Online] Available at: www.avert.org/professionals/hiv-around-world/global-response/funding [Accessed 22 March 2019].

Barnard, D., 2002. In the High Court of South Africa, Case no. 4138/98: The Global Politics of Access to Low-Cost AIDS Drugs in Poor Countries. *Kennedy Institute of Ethics Journal*, 12(2), pp. 159–174.

Barnett, A. & Blaikie, P., 1990. *AIDS in Africa: Its Present and Future Impact*. London: John Wiley and Co.

Barnett, A. & Whiteside, A., 2002. *AIDS in the Twenty-First Century: Disease and Globalization*. Hampshire: Palgrave MacMillan.

Barnett, T. & Prins, G., 2006. HIV/AIDS and Security: Fact, Fiction and Evidence – A Report to UNAIDS. *International Affairs*, 82, pp. 359–368.

Barnighausen, T., Bloom, D. & Humair, S., 2007. Human Resources for Treating HIV/AIDS: Needs, Capacities, and Gaps. *AIDS Patient Care*, 21, pp. 799–812.

Barro, J., 2014. *The Upshot*. [Online] Available at: www.nytimes.com/2014/11/17/upshot/aids-group-wages-lonely-fight-against-pill-to-prevent-hiv.html?abt=0002&abg=0 [Accessed 14 August 2015].

Basilico, M., et al., 2013. Health For All? Competing Theories and Geopolitics. In: P. Farmer, A. Kleinman, J. Kim & M. Basilico, eds. *Reimagining Global Health*. Berkeley and Los Angeles: University of California Press, pp. 74–110.

Bauman, Z., 1998. *Globalization: The Human Consequences*. Cambridge: Polity.

Bayer, R., 1991. Public Health Policy and the AIDS Epidemic: An End to HIV Exceptionalism? *New England Journal of Medicine*, 324, pp. 1500–1504.

Behrman, G., 2004. *The Invisible People*. New York: Free Press.

Bekker, L., et al., 2012. Southern African Guidelines for the Safe Use of Pre-Exposure Prophylaxis in Men Who Have Sex with Men Who Are At Risk For HIV Infection. *SAJHIVMED*, 13(2), pp. 40–55.

Bennet, S., et al., 2014. Policy Challenges Facing Integrated Case Management in Sub-Saharan Africa. *Tropical Medicine and International Health*, 19, pp. 872–882.

Berman, P., Gwatkin, D. & Burger, S., 1987. Community-Based Health Workers: Head Start or False Start Towards Health For All? *Social Science & Medicine*, 25, pp. 443–459.

Beukes, L., 2008. *Moxyland*. London: Angry Robot Publishers.

Beyrer, C., 2015. *Achieving Equity: The Imperative for Key Populations*. 7th International AIDS Conference, July 2015.

Bhutta, Z., Lassi, Z., Pariyo, G. & Huicho, L., 2010. *Global Experience of Community Health Workers for Delivery of Health Related Millenium Development Goals: A Systematic Review, Country Case Studies, and Recommendations for Integration into National Health Systems*. Geneva: WHO and Global Health Workforce Alliance.

Biehl, J., 2004. The Activist State: Global Pharmaceuticals, AIDS, and Citizenship in Brazil. *Social Text*, 22(3), pp. 105–132.

Biehl, J., 2007. *Will to Live. AIDS Therapies and the Politics of Survival*. Princeton and London: Princeton University Press.

Biehl, J. & Petryna, A., 2013. *When People Come First. Critical Studies in Global Health*. Princeton and Oxford: Princeton University Press.

Bond, P., 2000. *Elite Transition: From Apartheid to Neoliberalism in South Africa*. London: Pluto.

Boym, S., 2001. *The Future of Nostalgia*. New York: Basic Books.

Bowtell, B., 2007. *Applying the Paradox of Prevention: Eradicate HIV*, Griffith Review 17.

Brada, B., 2013. "Not Here": Making the Spaces and Subjects of "Global Health" in Botswana. *Culture, Medicine, and Psychiatry*, 35, pp. 285–312.

Burchardt, M., 2014. AIDS Activism in the Age of ARV Treatment in South Africa: Christianity, Resource Mobilization and the Meanings of Engagement. *Journal of Southern African Studies*, 40(1), pp. 59–74.

Burman, C., 2018. The Taming Wicked Problems Framework: A Plausible Biosocial Contribution to ending AIDS by 2030. *The Journal for Transdisciplinary Research in Southern Africa*, 14(1), pp. 1–12.

Butler, J., 1990. *Gender Trouble: Feminism and the Subversion of Identity*. New York: Routledge.

Butler, A., 2005. South Africa's HIV/AIDS Policy, 1994–2004: How Can It Be Explained? *African Affairs*, 104, pp. 591–614.

Castells, M., 1997. *The Power of Identity*. Malden: Blackwell.

Chambers, R., 2004. *Untimely Interventions. AIDS Writing, Testimonial, and the Rhetoric of Haunting*. Ann Arbor: University of Michigan Press.

Chazan, M., 2008. Surviving Politics and the Politics of Survival: Understanding Community Mobilization in South Africa. In: M. L. Foller & H. Thorn, eds. *The Politics of AIDS*. New York: Palgrave Macmillan, pp. 199–221.

Cheru, F., 2001. Overcoming Apartheid's Legacy: The Ascendancy of Neoliberalism in South Africa's Anti-Poverty Strategy. *Third World Quarterly*, 22, pp. 505–527.

Chin, J., 2006. *The AIDS Pandemic*. Oxford: Radcliffe Publishing.

Chirimuuta, R. & Chirimuuta, R., 1987. *AIDS, Africa and Racism*. Burton-on-Trent: Stanhope.

Cohen, L., 2005. The Kothi Wars: AIDS Cosmopolitanism and the Morality of Classification. In: M. Rivkin-Fish, A. Adams & S. Pigg, eds. *Sex in Development: Science, Sexuality and Morality in Global Perspectives*. Durham: Duke University Press, pp. 269–303.

Cohen, S., 2006. *Pharmanoia Coming to a Clinical Trial Near You*. [Online] Available at: www.slate.com/id/2136721/ [Accessed 12 September 2018].

Cohen, S. & Guthrie, T., 2014. *Financing the South African National Strategic Plan for HIV, STIs and TB 2012–2016*. Pretoria: SANAC.

Collins, J. & Rau, B., 2000. *AIDS in the Context of Development*. Geneva: UNRIDS Programme on Social Policy and Development.

Colvin, C., 2014. Evidence and AIDS Activism: HIV Scale-Up and the Contemporary Politics of Knowledge in Global Public Health. *Global Public Health*, 9(1–2), pp. 57–72.

Colvin, C. & Swartz, A., 2015. Extension Agents or Agents of Change? Community Health Workers and the Politics of Care Work in postapartheid South Africa. *Annals of Anthropological Practice*, 39(1), pp. 29–41.

Comaroff, J., 2007. Beyond Bare Life: AIDS, (Bio)Politics and the Neoliberal Order. *Public Culture*, 19(1), pp. 197–219.

Comaroff, J., 2010. Beyond Bare Life: AIDS, (Bio)Politics, and the Neoloberal Order. In: H. Dilger & U. Luig, eds. *Morality, Hope and Grief. Anthropologies of AIDS in Africa*. New York: Berghahn Books, pp. 21–42.

Comaroff, J. & Comaroff, J., 1999. *Civil Society and the Political Imagination in Africa: Critical Perspectives*. Chicago: Chicago University Press.

Connell, R., et al., 2018. Negotiating with the North: How Southern-tier Intellectual Workers Deal with the Global Economy of Knowledge. *The Sociological Review*, 66(1), pp. 41–57.

Cooper, H., Zimmerman, R. & McGinley, L., 2001. *AIDS Epidemic Puts Drug Firms in a Vise: Treatment vs. Profits*. [Online] Available at: www.wsj.com/articles/SB983487988418159849 [Accessed 12 December 2017].

Crane, J. T., 2013. *Scrambling For Africa. AIDS, Expertise, and the Rise of American Global Health Science*. Ithaca and London: Cornell University Press.

Cullinan, K. & Nkosi, S., 2015. *Health-e News: Stuck in a Limbo, Free State's Community Healthworkers Struggle to Get Their Jobs Back*. [Online] Available at: www.dailymaverick.co.za/article/2015-07-13-health-e-news-stuck-in-a-limbo-free-states-community-healthworkers-struggle-to-get-their-jobs-back/#.VpSpV18aLIU [Accessed 4 January 2016].

De Cock, K. M., Mbori-Ngacha, D. & Marum, E., 2002. Shadow on the Continent: Public Health and HIV/AIDS in Africa in the 21st Century. *Lancet*, 360, pp. 62–72.

de la Durantaye, L., 2005. The Exceptional Life of the State. Giorgio Agamben's State of Exception. *Genre*, XXXVIII, pp. 179–196.

De Wet, K., 2010. Les Trois Ages de la Santé Communautaire en Afrique du Sud. *Sciences Sociales et Santé*, 28, pp. 85–107.

De Wet, K., 2011. Redefining Volunteerism: The Rhetoric of Community Home-Based Care in (the Not So New) South Africa. *Community Development Journal*, 47(1), pp. 111–125.

Decoteau, C., 2013. *Ancestors and Antiretrovirals: The Biopolitics of HIV/AIDS in Post-Apartheid South Africa*. Chicago and London: University of Chicago Press.

Deghaye, N. & Whiteside, A., 2012. HIV Budgets Come Under Pressure. *The Mail & Guardian*, 12 September.

Department of Health, 2015. *National Health Insurance for South Africa. Towards Universal Health Coverage*, Pretoria: Department of Health.

Dixon, J. & Tameris, M., 2018. A Disease beyond Reach: Nurse Perspectives on the Past and Present of Tuberculosis in South Africa. *Anthropology Southern Africa*, 41(4), pp. 257–269.

Dworzanowski-Venter, B., 2008. 'Lazy Bugs, Homosexuals, Softies, and Dumb Fools': Exploring What It Means to Be a Male Emotional Labourer across Community-based AIDS Care Sites in Rural and Urban South Africa. *South African Review of Sociology*, 39(1), pp. 122–139.

Dworzanowski-Venter, B. & Smit, R., 2008. 'Most, They Don't Practice What They Preach': Exploring Personal Vulnerability and Risk Perceptions Amongst AIDS Caregivers in Ekurhuleni, South Africa. *South African Review of Sociology*, 39(1), pp. 65–82.

Eakle, R., Venter, F. & Rees, H., 2018. Pre-exposure Prohylaxis (PrEP) in an Era of Stalled HIV Prevention: Can it Change the Game? *Retrovirology*, 15(29), pp. 1–10.

Earth Institute, 2011. *One Million Community Health Workers: Task Force Report*. New York: Columbia University.

England, R., 2008. Writing Is on the Wall for UNAIDS. *British Medical Journal*, 336(1072), p. 1072.

Epstein, S., 1996. *Impure Science. AIDS, Activism, and the Politics of Knowledge*. Berkeley: University of California Press.

Epstein, H., 2007. *The Invisible Cure: Africa, the West, and the Fight against AIDS*. New York: Straus and Giroux.

Fallabela, L. S., Missana, S., Marilef, R. & Maurizi, M. R., 2009. *Writing and Publishing. Keys for Social Change*. Santiago: ESE. [Online] Available at: www.eseo.cl/public/doc/ESEO-workshop-Vietnam.pdf [Accessed 26 October 2015].

Farmer, P., 1999. *Infections and Inequalities. The Modern Plagues*. Berkeley: University of California Press.

Farmer, P., 2000. The Consumption of the Poor: Tuberculosis in the 21st Century. *Ethnography*, 1(2), pp. 183–216.

Farmer, P., Kim, J., Kleinman, A. & Basilico, M., 2013. Introduction: A Biosocial Approach to Global Health. In: P. Farmer, J. Kim, A. Kleinman & M. Basilico, eds. *Reimagining Global Health. An Introduction*. Berkeley and Los Angeles: University of California Press, pp. 1–14.

Farmer, P., Walton, D. & Tarter, L., 2000. Infections and Inequalities. *Global Change and Human Health*, 1(2), pp. 94–109.

Fassin, D., 2002. Embodied History. Uniqueness and Exemplarity of South African AIDS. *African Journal of AIDS Research*, 1, pp. 63–68.

Fassin, D., 2007. *When Bodies Remember. Experiences and Politics of AIDS in South Africa*. Berkeley: University of California Press.

Fassin, D., 2012a. *Humanitarian Reason. A Moral History of the Present*. Berkeley: University of California Press.

Fassin, D., 2012b. That Obscure Object of Global Health. In: M. C. Inhorn & E. Wentzell, eds. *Medical Anthropology at the Intersections: Histories, Activisms and Futures*. Durham: Duke University Press, pp. 95–115.

Feldberg, G., 1995. *Disease and Class: Tuberculosis and the Shaping of Modern North American Society*. New Brunswick: Rutgers University Press.

Fiedler, J., 2000. The Nepal National Vitamen a Program: Prototype to Emulate or Donor Enclave? *Health Policy Planning*, 15(2), pp. 145–156.

FIN24, 2019. Unemployment Rate Drops Marginally to 27.1% at End of 2018-Stats SA. Available at: www.fin24.com/Economy/unemployment-rate-drops-marginally-to-271-at-end-of-2018-stats-sa-20190212 [Accessed 12 February 2019].

Fourie, P. & Swart, C., 2014. South Africa's Future AIDS Governance: A Focused Elite Survey. *Development*, 56(4), pp. 511–517.

Frankenberg, R., 1986. Sickness as Cultural Performance: Drama, Trajectory, and Pilgramage Root Metaphors and the Making Social of Disease. *International Journal of Health Services*, 16, pp. 603–626.

Friedman, S. & Mottiar, S., 2004. *Rewarding Engagement? The Treatment Action Campaign and the Politics of HIV/AIDS*. Durban: University of KwaZulu Natal.

Friedman, S. & Mottiar, S., 2005. A Rewarding Engagement? The Treatment Action Campaign and the Politics of HIV/AIDS. *Politics & Society*, 33(4), pp. 511–561.

Fukayama, F., 2014. At the 'End of History' Still Stands Democracy. *The Wall Street Journal*, 6 June, pp. 6–14.

Garrett, L., 2012. Money or Die. A Watershed Moment for Global Public Health. *Foreign Affairs*, 6 March. Available at: www.foreignaffairs.com/articles/2012-03-06/money-or-die [Accessed 25 June 2019].

Geffen, N., 2010. *Debunking Delusions. The Inside Story of the Treatment Action Campaign*. Pretoria: Jacana Media.

Geffen, N. & Gonsalves, G., 2008. In Defence of Rational AIDS Activism. How Irrationality of Act-Up Paris and Others is Risking the Health of People with HIV or at Risk of HIV Infection. *The Southern African Journal of HIV Medicine*, 9(2), pp. 12–17.

Gilmore, B. & McAuliffe, E., 2013. Effectiveness of Community Health Workers Delivering Preventive Interventions for Maternal and Child Health in Low-and Middle-Income Countries: A Systemic Review. *BMC Public Health*, 13(1), p. 847.

Gilson, L., Walt, G., Heggenhougen, K., et al., 1989. National Community Health Programs: How Can They be Strengthened? *Journal for Public Health Policy*, 10(4), pp. 518–532.

Gonsalves, G. & Staley, P., 2014. Panic, Paranoia and Public Health – The AIDS Epidemic's Lessons for Ebola. *The New England Journal of Medicine*, 371(25), pp. 2348–2349.

Gore, A., 2000. *Remarks as Prepared for Delivery by Vice President Al Gore for the UN Security Council Session on AIDS in Africa*. Washington: United Nations Security Council.

Govender, P., 2012. *US Hands More Control to South Africa in Its AIDS Fight*. [Online] Available at: www.reuters.com/article/2012/08/07/us-clinton-safricaaids-aids-idUSBRE8760ZU20120807 [Accessed 7 September 2015].

Grady, D., 2001. Generic Medicine for AIDS Raises New Set of Concerns. *New York Times*, 24 April.

Grebe, E., 2011. The Treatment Action Campaign's Struggle for AIDS Treatment in South Africa: Coalition Building through Networks. *Journal of Southern African Studies*, 37(4), pp. 849–868.

Green, A., 2015. *Community Health Workers Back in Court*. [Online] Available at: http://mg.co.za/article/2015-01-28-community-health-workers-back-in-court [Accessed 4 January 2016].

Green, J., Thorp Basilico, M., Kim, H. & Farmer, P., 2013. Colonial Medicine and Its Legacies. In: P. Farmer, J. Kim, A. Kleinman & M. Basilico, eds. *Reimagining Global Health. An Introduction*. Berkeley and Los Angeles: University of California Press, pp. 33–73.

Grewal, I. & Kaplan, C., 1994. *Scattered Hegemonies: Postmodernity and Transnational Feminist Practice*. Minneapolis: University of Minnesota Press.

Haines, A., Sanders, D., Lehman, U., et al., 2007. Achieving Child Survival Goals: Potential Contribution of Community Health Workers. *Lancet*, 369(9579), pp. 2121–2131.

Harper, I., 2006. Anthropology, DOTS and Understanding Tuberculosis in Nepal. *Journal of Biosocial Science*, 38(1), pp. 57–67.

Harries, A., et al., 2001. Preventing Antiretroviral Anarchy in Sub-Saharan Africa. *Lancet*, 358(9279), pp. 410–414.

Harrington, A., 2005. *Modern Social Theory. An Introduction*. Oxford: Oxford University Press.

Harrington, M., 2010. From HIV to Tuberculosis and Back Again: A Tale of Activism in 2 Pandemics. *Clinical Infectious Diseases*, 50(3), pp. S260–S266.

Health E-News, 2015. *Free State Protest for Community Health Workers*. [Online] Available at: www.health-e.org.za/2015/04/01/free-state-protest-for-community-health-workers/ [Accessed 4 January 2016].

Herbert, B., 2001. In America; Refusing to Save Africans. *The New York Times*, 11 June.

Heywood, M., 2003. Preventing Mother-to-Child HIV Transmission in South Africa: Background, Strategies and Outcomes of the Treatment Action Campaign Case against the Minister of Health. *South African Journal of Human Rights*, 19, pp. 278–315.

Heywood, M., 2009. South Africa's Treatment Action Campaign: Combining Law and Social Mobilization to Realize the Right to Health. *Journal of Human Rights Practice*, 1(1), pp. 14–36.

Hlatshwayo, M., 2018. The New Struggles of Precarious Workers in South Africa: Nascent Organizational Responses of Community Health Workers. *Review of African Political Economy*, 45(157), pp. 378–392.

Hodes, R. & Morrell, R., 2018. Incursions from the Epicenter: Southern Theory, Social Science and the Global HIV Research Domain. *African Journal of AIDS Research*, 17(1), pp. 22–31.

Human Sciences Research Council, 2015. *The People Living with HIV Stigma Index: South Africa 2014*, Pretoria: HSRC.

Hunt, N., 1997. *Among AIDS Derivatives in Africa*. [Online] Available at: https://quod.lib.umich.edu/j/jii/4750978.0004.301/--among-aids-derivatives-in-africa?rgn=main;view=fulltext [Accessed 14 August 2018].

ICASO, 2015. *Discussion Paper: Regional Concept Note Development in the Global Fund's (New) Funding Model: Observations from the First Round of Regional Concept Notes*, ICASO.

INCIDENCE, 2014. *Incidence. No-Nonsense Evidence-based HIV Prevention Approach*. [Online] Available at: www.incidence0.org/2014/11/13/pre-exposure-prophylaxis-latest-fad-or-a-drive-for-change/ [Accessed 14 August 2015].

Ingram, A., 2013. After the Exception: HIV/AIDS beyond Salvation and Scarcity. *Antipode*, 45(2), pp. 436–454.

International AIDS Vaccine Initiative, 2017. *IAVI and Oxford University Initiate Africa-Europe Partnership to Develop an AIDS Vaccine*. [Online] Available at: www.iavi.org/newsroom/press-releases/2017/iavi-and-oxford-university-initiate-africa-europe-partnership-to-develop-an-aids-vaccine [Accessed 4 March 2019].

International Labor Organization, n.d. *Decent Work*. [Online] Available at: www.ilo.org/global/topics/decent-work/lang--en/index.htm [Accessed 29 September 2018].

IRIN, 2012. *HIV/AIDS. New Ways to Fund the Fight.* [Online] Available at: www. irinnews.org/report/95946/hiv-aids-new-ways-to-fund-the-fight [Accessed 4 September 2015].

Irwin, A., 1995. *Citizen Science. A Study of People, Expertise and Sustainable Development.* London: Routledge.

Jolly, R., 2010. *Cultured Violence: Narrative, Social Suffering and Engendering Human Rights.* Liverpool: Liverpool University Press.

Jungar, K. & Oinas, E., 2010. A Feminist Struggle? South African HIV Activism as Feminist Politics. *Journal of International Women's Studies,* 11(4), pp. 177–191.

Jungar, K. & Oinas, E., 2011. Beyond Agency and Victimization: Re-reading HIV and AIDS in African Contexts. *Social Dynamics,* 37(2), pp. 248–262.

Kates, J., et al., 2011. *Financing the Response to AIDS In low- and Middle- Income Countries: International Assistance from Donor Governments in 2010.* Washington: Kaiser Family Foundation and Joint United Nations Program on HIV/AIDS.

King, N., 2002. Security, Disease Commerce. Ideologies of Postcolonial Global Health. *Social Studies of Science,* 32(5–6), pp. 763–789.

Kingori, P. & Sariola, S., 2015. Museum of Failed HIV Research. *Anthropology & Medicine,* 22(3), pp. 213–216.

Kippax, S., Stephenson, N., Parker, R. & Aggleton, P., 2013. Between Individual Agency and Structure in HIV Prevention: Understanding the Middle Ground of Social Practice. *American Journal of Public Health,* 103(8), pp. 1367–1375.

Klein, N., 2007. *The Shock Doctrine. The Rise of Disaster Capitalism.* London: Penguin.

Kleinman, A., 2010. Four Social Theories for Global Health. *Lancet,* 375, pp. 1518–1519.

Kleinman, A., Das, V. & Lock, M., 1997. *Social Suffering.* Berkeley: University of California Press.

Kleinman, A. & Kleinman, J., 1997. The Appeal of Experience; The Dismay of Images: Cultural Appropriations of Suffering in Our Times. In: A. Kleinman, V. Das & M. Lock, eds. *Social Suffering.* Berkeley: University of California Press, pp. 1–24.

Knight, L., 2006. *UNAIDS. The First Ten Years, 1996–2006.* Geneva: UNAIDS.

Kok, M., et al., 2015. How Does Context Influence Performance of Community Health Workers in Low- and Middle-Income Countries? Evidence from the Literature. *Health Research Policy and Systems,* 13(1), p. 13.

Koplan, J., et al., 2009. Towards a Common Definition of Global Health. *The Lancet,* 373(9679), pp. 1993–1995.

Kopp, C., 2002. *The New Era of AIDS. HIV and Medicine in Times of Transition.* Dordrecht: Kluwer Academic Publishers.

Lakoff, A., 2005. *Pharmaceutical Reason. Knowledge and Value in Global Psychiatry.* Cambridge: Cambridge University Press.

Lakoff, A., 2010. Two Regimes of Global Health. *Humanity: An International Journal of Human Rights, Humanitarianism, and Development,* 1(1), pp. 59–79.

Lather, P., 2002. Postbook: Working the Ruins of Feminist Ethnography. *Signs,* 27(1), pp. 199–227.

Lehmann, U., Van Damme, W., Barten, F. & Sanders, D., 2009. Task Shifting: The Answer to the Human Resources Crisis in Africa? *Human Resources for Health,* 7, p. 49.

Leon, N., et al., 2015. The Role of "Hidden" Community Volunteers in Community-Based Health Service Delivery Platforms: Examples from sub-Saharan Africa. *Global Health Action,* 8, p. 272114.

Lewin, S., et al., 2012. Lay Health Workers in Primary and Community Health Care for Maternal and Child Health and the Management of Infectious Diseases. *Cochrane Database Systematic Review*. [Online] Available at: https://www.cochranelibrary.com/cdsr/doi/10.1002/14651858.CD004015.pub2/epdf/full [Accessed 25 June 2019].

Loewenstein, A., 2016. *Disaster Capitalism. Making a Killing out of Catastrophe*. New York: Verso Books.

London, L. & Schneider, H., 2012. Globalisation and Health Inequalities: Can a Human Rights Paradigm Create Space for Civil Society Action? *Social Science & Medicine*, 74, pp. 6–13.

Maartens, G., 2015. *The Next Generation ARVs. What can we Look Forward to?* Durban, 7th South African AIDS Conference, July 2015.

Maes, K., 2015. "Volunteers are not paid because they are Priceless": Community Health Worker Capacities and Values in an AIDS Treatment Intervention in Urban Ethiopia. *Medical Anthropology Quarterly*, 29(1), pp. 97–115.

Malan, M., 2014a. *TAC Community Health Care Workers Arrested in Free State*. [Online] Available at: http://mg.co.za/article/2014-07-10-tac-community-healthcare-workers-arrested-in-free-state [Accessed 4 January 2016].

Malan, M., 2014b. *Why Policy is Failing Community Health Workers*. [Online] Available at: http://mg.co.za/article/2014-09-04-why-policy-is-failing-community-health-workers [Accessed 4 January 2016].

Malan, M., 2015. Exposé Spurs Flurry of Activity, But Problems Remain. *The Mai & Guardian*, 12–18 June, p. 26.

Marais, H., 2001. *South Africa, Limits to Change: The Political Economy of Transition*. London: Zed Books.

Marazzo, J., et al., 2015. Tenofovir-Based Pre-Exposure Prohylaxis for HIV Infection among African Women. *The New England Journal of Medicine*, 372(6), pp. 509–518.

Matebeni, Z., 2015. *Silencing Sex: Lesbian and Bisexual Women beyond the Margins*, 7th International AIDS Conference, Durban July 2015.

Mayberry, A. & Baker, T., 2011. Lessons from a Brazilian-US Cooperative Health Program: The Serviço Especial de Saude publica. *Public Health Report*, 126, pp. 276–282.

Mbali, M., 2004. AIDS Discourses and the South African State. Government Denialism and Post-apartheid AIDS Policy-making. *Transformation*, 54, pp. 104–122.

Mbali, M., 2005. The Treatment Action Campaign and the History of Rights-Based, Patient-Driven HIV/AIDS Activism in South Africa. In: P. Jones & K. Stokke, eds. *Democratizing Development: The Politics of Socio-Economic Rights in South Africa*. Leiden: Martinus Nijhoff, pp. 213–243.

Mbali, M., 2013. *South African AIDS Activism and Global Health Politics*. New York: Palgrave Macmillan.

Mbeki, T., 2001. *ZK Matthews Memorial Lecture*. Fort Hare University.

Mbembe, A., 2001. *On the Postcolony*. Johannesburg: Wits University Press.

Mbembe, A., 2002. African Modes of Self Writing. *Public Culture*, 14(1), pp. 239–273.

Mbembe, A., 2003. Necropolitics. *Public Culture*, 15(1), pp. 11–40.

McGoey, L., 2015. *No Such Thing as a Free Gift. The Gates Foundation and the Price of Philanthropy*. New York: Verso Books.

McNeil, M. C., 2005. Introduction: Postcolonial Technoscience (Special Edition). *Science as Culture*, 14 (2), pp. 105–122.

McNeil, D., 2015a. *The New York Times.* [Online] Available at: www.nytimes.com/2015/02/05/health/failed-trial-in-africa-raises-questions-about-how-to-test-hiv-drugs.html?_r=0 [Accessed 15 August 2015].

McNeil, D., 2015b. *US Push for Abstinence in Africa is seen as Failure against HIV.* [Online] Available at: www.nytimes.com/2015/02/27/health/american-hiv-battle-in-africa-said-to-falter.html [Accessed 12 December 2017].

Mindry, D., 2008. Neoliberalism, Activism, and HIV/AIDS in Postapartheid South Africa. *Social Text*, 26(1), pp. 75–93.

Moletsane, R., 2014. *Nostalgia AIDS Review 2013*, University of Pretoria: Centre for the Study of AIDS.

Montgomery, C., 2015. "HIV has a Woman's Face': Vaginal Microbicides and a Case of Ambiguous Failure. *Anthropology & Medicine*, 22(3), pp. 250–262.

Msomi, N., 2019. *Making the Sale: Re-branding the HIV Prevention Pill for Women.* [Online] Available at: mailandguardian.evlink1.net/servlet/link/6026/976179/84083780/5052984 [Accessed 29 March 2019].

MSF, 2009. *HIV/AIDS Treatment in Developing Countries: The Battle for Long-term Survival has just begun.* Geneva: Médecins Sans Frontières.

Mudimbe, V., 1988. *The Invention of Africa: Gnosis, Philosophy and the Order of Knowledge.* Bloomington and Indianapolis: Indiana University Press.

Mundeva, H., Snyder, J., Ngilangwa, D. & Kaida, A., 2018. Ethics of Task Shifting in the Health Workforce: Exploring the Role of Community Health Workers in HIV Service Delivery in Low- and Middle-Income Countries. *BMC Medical Ethics*, 19(71).

Mwai, G., et al., 2013. Role and Outcomes of Community Health Workers in HIV Care in sub-Saharan Africa: A Systemic Review. *Journal of the International AIDS Society*, 16, p. 18586.

Mykhalovskiy, E. & Rosengarten, M., 2009a. Editorial. HIV/AIDS in its Third Decade: Renewed Critique in Social and Cultural Analysis – An Introduction. *Social Theory & Health*, 7, pp. 187–195.

Mykhalovskiy, E. & Rosengarten, M., 2009b. Commentaries on the Nature of Social and Cultural Research: Interviews on HIV/AIDS with Judy Auerbach, Susan Kippax, Steven Epstein, Didier Fassin, Barry Adam, and Dennis Altman. *Social Theory & Health*, 7, pp. 284–304.

Naidu, T., Sliep, Y. & Dageid, W., 2012. The Social Construction of Identity in HIV/AIDS Home-based Care Volunteers in Rural KwaZulu-Natal, South Africa. *SAHARA – J: Journal of Social Aspects of HIV/AIDS*, 9(2), pp. 113–126.

Navario, P., et al., 2012. *Special Report on the State of HIV/AIDS in South Africa.* [Online] Available at: www.cssr.uct.ac.za/pub/journal-article/2012/special-report-state-hivaids-south-africa [Accessed 2 September 2015].

Nelkin, D., 1995. Science Controversies: The Dynamic of Public Disputes in the United States. In: S. Jasanhoff, G. E. Markle, J. C. Petersen & T. Pinch, eds. *Handbook of Science and Technology Studies*. Thousand Oaks: Sage Publications, pp. 444–456.

Nguyen, V., 2004. Antiretroviral Globalism, Biopolitics, and Therapeutic Citizenship. In: S. J. Collier & A. Ong, eds. *Global Assemblages: Technology, Politics, and Ethics as Anthropological Problems*. Malden: Blackwell Publishers, pp. 124–144.

Nguyen, V., 2010. *The Republic of Therapy: Triage and Sovereignty in West Africa's Time of AIDS.* Durham and London: Duke University Press.

Nguyen, V. & Peschard, K., 2003. Anthropology, Inequality, and Disease: A Review. *Annual Review of Anthropology*, 32, pp. 447–474.

Nguyen, V. K. & Sama, M. T., 2008. Determinants of HIV Transmission: Lessons from Africa. In: M. T. Sama & V. Nguyen, eds. *Governing Health Systems in Africa*. Senegal: CODESRIA, pp. 237–355.

Olesen, T., 2006. 'In the Court of Public Opinion': Transnational Problem Construction in the HIV/AIDS Medicine Access Campaign, 1998–2001. *International Sociology*, 21(5), pp. 5–30.

Olick, J., 2007. *The Politics of Regret. On Collective Memory and Historical Responsibility*. New York: Routledge.

Oomman, N., Bernstein, M. & Rosenzweig, S., 2007. *Following the Funding for HIV/AIDS: A Comparative Analysis of PEPFAR, the Global Fund and World Bank MAP*, Washington: Center for Global Development.

Oppenheimer, G. M. & Bayer, R., 2009. The Rise and Fall of AIDS Exceptionalism. *American Medical Association Journal of Ethics*, 11(12), pp. 988–992.

Over, M., 2008. *Prevention Failure: The Ballooning Entitlement Burden of US Global AIDS Treatment Spending and What To Do About It*. Washington: Center for Global Development.

Owen, T., 2018. Twenty One Years of HIV/AIDS Medicines in the Newspaper: Patents, Protests, and Philantropy. *Media, Culture & Society*, 40(1), pp. 75–93.

Packard, R., 2016. *A History of Global Health. Interventions into the Lives of Other Peoples*. Baltimore: Johns Hopkins University Press.

Pandolfi, M., 2000. Une souveraineté mouvante et supracoloniale: L'industrie humanitaire dans les Balkans. *Multitudes*, 3, pp. 97–105.

Parker, R., 2011. Grassroots Activism, Civil Society Mobilization, and the Politics of the Global HIV/AIDS Epidemic. *Brown Journal of World Affairs*, XVII(II), pp. 21–37.

Patton, C., 1990a. Inventing "African AIDS". *New Formations*, 10, pp. 25–39.

Patton, C., 1990b. *Inventing AIDS*. New York: Routledge.

Patton, C., 2002. *Globalizing AIDS (Theory out of Bounds)*. Minneapolis: University of Minnesota Press.

Penfold, E., 2015. *The Securitization of HIV/AIDS in Post-Cold War Era: Discursive Shift in International Relations*. Durban: Association for Social Sciences and Humanities for the Study of HIV/AIDS, June 2015.

Perry, H., 2013. *A Brief History of Community Health Worker Programs*. s.l.: s.n.

Perry, H., Hodgins, S., Crigler, L. & LeBan, K., 2013. *Community Health Worker Relationships with Other Parts of the Health System*. [Online] Available at: www.mchip. net/sites/default/files/mchipfiles/11_CHW_HealthSystems.pdf [Accessed 25 June 2019].

Perry, H. & Zulliger, R., 2012. *How Effective Are Community Health Workers? An Overview of Current Evidence with Recommendations for Strengthening Community Health Worker Programs to Accelerate Progress in Achieving the Health-Related Millennium Goals*. Baltimore: Johns Hopkins School of Public Health.

Perry, H., Zulliger, R. & Rogers, M., 2014. Community Health Workers in Low- and High-Income Countries: An Overview of Their History, Recent Evolution, and Current Effectiveness. *Annual Review of Public Health*, 35, pp. 399–421.

Petryna, A., 2002. *Life Exposed: Biological Citizens after Chernobyl*. Princeton: Princeton University Press.

Pharaoh, R. & Schonteich, M., 2003. *AIDS, Security, and Governance in Southern Africa. Exploring the Impact. Occasional Paper No 65*. Pretoria: Institute for Security Studies.

Pigg, S., 2013. On Sitting and Doing: Ethnography as Action in Global Health. *Social Science & Medicine*, 99, pp. 127–134.

Pillay, Y. & Barron, P., 2011. [Online] Available at: www.phasa.org.za/articles/the-implementation-of-phc-re-engineering-in-south-africa.html [Accessed 3 December 2015].

Piot, P., 2008. *AIDS: Exceptionalism Revisited (Speech at London School of Economics and Political Science)*. London: UNAIDS.

Pisani, E., 2008. *The Wisdom of Whores: Bureaucrats, Brothels and the Business of AIDS*. London: Granta.

PlusNews, 2009. *Global AIDS Funding at "Dangerous Turning Point"*. [Online] Available at: www.plusnews.org/Report.aspx?Reportld+8690 [Accessed 18 September 2018].

Pogge, T. W., 2002. Moral Universalism and Global Economic Justice. *Politics, Philosophy & Economics*, 1(1), pp. 29–58.

Popp, D. & Fisher, J., 2002. First, Do No Harm: A Call for Emphasizing Adherence and HIV Prevention Interventions in Active Antiretroviral Therapy Programs in the Developing World. *AIDS*, 16(4), pp. 676–678.

Posel, D., 2000. A Mania for Measurement: Statistics and Statecraft in Modern South Africa. In: S. Dubow, ed. *Science and Society in Southern Africa*. Manchester and New York: Manchester University Press, pp. 116–137.

Powers, T., 2017. Knowlegde Practices, waves and verticality: Tracing HIV/AIDS Activism from Late Apartheid to the Present in South Africa. *Critique of Anthropology*, 37(1), pp. 27–46.

Rabinow, P., 1996. *Artificiality and Enlightenment: From Sociobiology to Biosociality. Essays on the Anthropology of Reason*. Princeton: Princeton University Press.

Race, K., 2001. The Undetectable Crisis: Changing Technologies of Risk. *Sexualities*, 4(2), pp. 167–189.

Ramaphosa, C., 2015. *Plenary Adress*. Durban: 7th South African AIDS Conference.

Raphael, Y., Kanyeemba, B., Yola, N. & Robinson, A., 2015. *AVAC*. [Online] Available at: www.avac.org/blog/south-african-aids-activists-demand-prep-now [Accessed 15 August 2015].

Redfield, P., 2012. Bioexpectations: Life Technologies as Humanitarian Goods. *Public Culture*, 24(166), pp. 157–184.

Republic of South Africa, 2017. *Let Our Actions Count: South Africa's National Strategic Plan for HIV, TB and STIs 2017–2022*. Pretoria: South Africa.

Reynolds, L. J., 2014. 'Low-Hanging Fruit': Counting and Accounting for Children in PEPFAR-Funded HIV/AIDS Programmes in South Africa. *Global Public Health*, 9(1–2), pp. 124–143.

Rifkin, S., 2008. Community Health Workers. In: W. Kirch, ed. *Encyclopedia of Public Health*. Berlin: Springer, pp. 773–781.

Robertson, R., 1992. *Globalization: Social Theory and Global Culture*. London: Sage.

Robins, S., 2004. 'Long live Zachy, long live': AIDS Activism, Science and Citizenship after Apartheid. *Journal of Southern African Studies*, 30(3), pp. 651–672.

Robins, S., 2005. *From 'Medical Miracles' to Normal(ised) Medicine: AIDS Treatment, Activism and Citizenship in the UK and South Africa*. Brighton: Institute of Development Studies Working Paper 252.

Robins, S. & von Lieres, B., 2004. Remaking Citizenship, Unmaking Marginalization: The Treatment Action Campaign in Post-Apartheid South Africa. *Canadian Journal of African Studies*, 38(3), pp. 575–586.

Rose, N., 2007. *The Politics of Life Itself. Biomedicine, Power, and Subjectivity in the Twenty-First Century.* Princeton: Princeton University Press.

Rose, N. & Novas, C., 2004. Biological Citizenship. In: A. Ong & S. Collier, eds. *Blackwell Companion to Global Anthropology.* Oxford: Blackwell.

Rosengarten, M., 2010. *HIV Interventions. Biomedicine and the Traffic between Information and Flesh.* Seattle: University of Washington Press.

Rosenthal, E., et al., 2010. Community Health Workers: Part of the Solution. *Health Affairs*, 29(7), pp. 1338–1342.

Rottenburg, R., 2009. Social and Public Experiments and New Figurations of Science and Politics in Postcolonial Africa. *Postcolonial Studies*, 12(4), pp. 423–440.

Runciman, C., 2015. The Decline of the Anti-privatisation Forum in the Midst of South Africa's 'Rebellion of the Poor'. *Current Sociology*, 63(7), pp. 961–979.

Rushton, S. & Williams, O., 2011. Private Actors in Global Health Governance. In: S. Rushton & O. Williams, eds. *Partnerships and Foundations in Global Health Governance.* London: Palgrave MacMillan, pp. 1–28.

Sahoo, S., 2010. AIDS Funding Flat-Lining, Groups Complain. *Inter Press Service News Agency*, 12 March.

Sama, M. & Nguyen, V., 2008. *Governing Health Systems in Africa.* Senegal: CODESRIA.

Scheper-Hughes, N., 1994. An Essay: AIDS and the Social Body. *Social Science & Medicine,* 39(7), pp. 991–1003.

Schneider, H., 2002. On the Fault-Line: The Politics of AIDS Policy Implementation in Contemporary South Africa. *African Studies*, 61, pp. 145–167.

Schneider, H., 2019. The Governance of National Community Health Worker Programmes in Low- and Middle-Income Countries: An Empirically Based Framework of Governance Principles, Purposes and Tasks. *International Journal of Health Policy and Management*, 8(1), pp. 18–27.

Schneider, H., et al., 2015. The Challenges of Reshaping Disease Specific and Care-Oriented Community Based Services towards Comprehensive Goals: A Situation Appraisal in the Western Cape Province, South Africa. *BMC Health Services Research*, 15(1), p. 436.

Schneider, H., Okello, D. & Lehmann, U., 2016. The Global Pendulum Swing towards Community Health Workers in Low- and Middle-income Countries: A Scoping Review of Trends, Geographical Distribution and Programmatic Orientations, 2005–2014. *Human Resources for Health*, 14(1), p. 65.

Schneider, H. & Nxumalo, N., 2017. Leadership and Governance of Community Health Worker Programmes at Scale: A Cross Case Analysis of Provincial Implementation in South Africa. *International Journal of Equity in Health*, 16(72), pp. 1–12.

Schneider, H. & Stein, J., 2001. Implementing AIDS Policy in Post-Apartheid South Africa. *Social Science & Medicine*, 52, pp. 723–731.

Schülenk, U., 2004. Professional Responsibilities of Biomedical Scientists in Public Discourse. *Journal of Medical Ethics*, 30, pp. 53–60.

Schwartländer, B., Stover, J., Hallett, T., et al., 2011. Towards an Improved Investment Approach for an Effective Response to HIV/AIDS. *The Lancet*, 377, pp. 2031–2041.

Section, 27, 2015. [Online] Available at: http://section27.org.za/2015/10/free-state-chws-to-appeal-shocking-judgement/ [Accessed 5 May 2017].

SECTION, 27, 2018. *WIPO Conference an Insult to People Who Died of AIDS.* [Online] [Accessed 17 February 2019].

Seidman, G., 1999. Is South Africa Different? Sociological Comparisons and Theoretical Contributions from the Land of Apartheid. *Annual Review of Sociology*, 25, pp. 419–440.

Selenko, E., Makikangas, A. & Stride, C., 2017. Does Job Insecurity Threaten who you are? Introducing a Social Identity Perspective to Explain Well-being and Performance Consequences of Job Insecurity. *Journal of Organizational Behavior*, 38, pp. 856–875.

Smith, L., 2012. *Decolonizing Methodologies: Research and Indigenous Peoples*. 2nd Edition. London: Zed Books.

Smith, J. H. & Whiteside, A., 2010. The History of AIDS Exceptionalism. *Journal of the International AIDS Society*, 13(48), pp. 1–8.

South African Government News Agency, 2019. *Increased Allocations in Grants, Education and Health*. [Online] Available at: www.treasury.gov.za/documents/national%20budget/2019/ene/FullENE.pdf [Accessed 13 March 2019].

Steinberg, J., 2007. *South Africa: Anthropology of Low Expectations*. [Online]

Steinberg, J., 2008. *Three-Letter Plague. A Young Man's Journey through a Great Epidemic*. London: Penguin Books.

Steinberg, J., 2016. Re-examining the Early Years of Anti-Retroviral Treatment in South Africa: A Taste for Medicine. *African Affairs*, 116(462), pp. 60–79.

Stephens, J., 2015. *NSP Review. HIV and Human Rights: The Right to Protest*. [Online] Available at: www.nspreview.org/2015/10/22/hiv-and-human-rights-the-right-to-protest/ [Accessed 4 January 2016].

TAC (Treatment Action Campaign), 2018. *State of Provincial Healthcare Sector. Spotlight on Free State*. [Online] Available at: https://tac.org.za/files/tac-fs-state-of-health-report-may-2018.pdf/ [Accessed 26 November 2018].

Tamale, E., 2011. *African Sexualities. A Reader*. Cape Town: Pambazuka Press.

Tarrow, S., 1994. *Power in Movement*. Cambridge: Cambridge University Press.

Tembo, J., 2018. Mbembe at the Lekgotla of Foucault's Self-styling and African Identity. *Phronimon*, 19(2121), pp. 1–17.

t'Hoen, E., Berger, J., Calmy, A., et al., 2011. Driving a Decade of Change: HIV/AIDS, Patents and Access to Medicines for all. *AIDS Society*, 14(15), pp. 1–12.

Thom, A. & Heywood, M., 2016. South Africa's Health System is ill but the Minister is not the Cause. *Business Live*, 11 December.

Trafford, Z., Swartz, A. & Colvin, C., 2018. "Contract to Volunteer": South African Community Health Worker Mobilization for better Labor Protection. *New Solutions: A Journal of Environmental and Occupational Health Policy*, 27(4), pp. 648–666.

Treatment Action Campaign & Section 27, 2016a. Spotlight. AIDS Durban 2000–2016. Available at: http://section27.org.za/wp-content/uploads/2017/02/000-spotlight-15-web.pdf/ [Accessed 2 December 2018].

Treatment Action Campaign & Section 27, 2016b. *Victory at last for #BohpeloHouse94: Long live Democracy and the Right to Protest*. [Online] Available at: https://tac.org.za/news/victory-at-last-for-bophelohouse94-long-live-democracy-and-the-right-to-protest/ [Accessed 8 October 2018].

Treichler, P., 1987. AIDS, Homophobia, and Biomedical Discourse: An Epidemic of Signification. *AIDS: Cultural Analysis/ Cultural Activism*, 43, pp. 31–70.

Treichler, P., 1989. AIDS and HIV Infection in the Third World: A First World Chronicle. In: B. Kruger & P. Mariani, eds. *Remaking History*. Seattle: Bay Press, pp. 31–86.

Treichler, P., 1999. *How to Have Theory in an Epidemic. Cultural Chronicles of AIDS*. Durham: Duke University Press.

UNAIDS, 2008. *UNAIDS: The First 10 Years.* Geneva, Switzerland: UNAIDS.

UNAIDS, 2009. *Joint Action for Results. UN Outcomes Framework 2009–2011.* Geneva: UNAIDS.

UNAIDS, 2013. *Global Report. UNAIDS Report on the Global AIDS Epidemic 2013.* Geneva: UNAIDS.

UNAIDS, 2014a. *90:90:90 An Ambitious Treatment Target to Help End the AIDS Epidemic.* Geneva: UNAIDS.

UNAIDS, 2014b. *Fast-Track. Ending the AIDS Epidemic by 2030.* Geneva: UNAIDS.

UNAIDS, 2015a. *Staying Ahead of the AIDS Epidemic in South Africa.* Geneva: UNAIDS.

UNAIDS, 2015b. *UNAIDS Announces that the Goal of 15 Million People on Life-saving HIV Treatment by 2015 Has Been Met Nine Months ahead of Schedule.* Geneva: UNAIDS.

UNAIDS, 2016. *Prevention Gap Report.* Geneva: Joint United Nations Program on HIV/AIDS.

UNAIDS & World Bank, 2009. *The Global Economic Crisis and HIV Prevention and Treatment Programmes: Vulnerabilities and Impact.* Geneva: UNAIDS & World Bank.

US National Intelligence Council, 2000. *The Global Infectious Disease Threat and its Implications for the United States of America.* Washington.

Van der Straten, A., et al., 2014. Perspectives on Use of Oral and Vaginal Antitretrovirals for HIV Prevention: The Voice C Qualitative Study in Johannesburg, South Africa. *Journal of the International AIDS Society,* 17 (Supplement 2).

Van der Vliet, V., 2001. AIDS: Losing 'The New Struggle'? *Daedalus,* 130(1), p. 155.

Van der Wal, R. & Loutfi, D., 2017. Pre-exposure Prophylaxis for HIV Prevention in East and Southern Africa. *Canadian Journal of Public Health,* 180(5–6), pp. e653–645.

Van Ginneken, N., Lewin, S. & Berridge, V., 2010. The Emergence of Community Health Worker Programmes in the Late Apartheid Era in South Africa: An Historical Analysis. *Social Science & Medicine,* 71, pp. 1110–1118.

Van Niekerk, A. A., 2014. Three Ethical Issues in the Development of Public Genetic Health Policies in Africa. *AIDS & Clinical Research,* 5, p. 399.

Van Pletzen, E., Zulliger, R., Moshabela, M. & Schneider, H., 2013. The Size, Characteristics and Partnership Networks of the Health-Related Non-Profit Sector in Three Regions of South Africa: Implications of Changing Primary Health Care Policy for Community-Based Care. *Health Policy and Planning,* 29, pp. 1–11.

Van Wyk, A. & Brodie, N., 2015. Crisis? What Crisis? Africa Check Tests Free State Health Claims. *The Mail & Guardian,* 12–18 June, pp. 26–27.

Venter, F., 2016. "The End of AIDS" Tune is Premature and Dangerous. In: *Treatment Action Campaign & Section 27. AIDS Durban 2000–2016.* Johannesburg: Treatment Action Campaign & Section 27, pp. 11–18.

Visual AIDS, 2014. *Your Nostalgia is Killing Me. Catalyst for Conversation about AIDS and Visual Culture.* [Online] Available at: www.visualaids.org/events/detail/your-nostalgia-is-killing-me-a-catalyst-for-conversation-about-aids-and-vis [Accessed 9 November 2015].

Walsh, J. A. & Warren, K. S., 1979. Selective Primary Health Care: An Interim Strategy for Disease Control in Developing Countries. *New England Journal of Medicine,* 301(18), p. 967.

Watney, S., 1989. Missionary Positions: AIDS, 'Africa', and Race. *Critical Quarterly,* 31(3), pp. 45–62.

Werner, D., 1977. [Online] Available at: www.healthwrights.org/content/articles/lackey_or_liberator.htm [Accessed 12 December 2018].

Whitaker, R., 2014. *The BMJ*. [Online] Available at: http://blogs.bmj.com/bmj/2014/11/07/rupert-whitaker-a-pill-for-risky-sex-another-step-on-the-road-to-a-pill-for-bad-housing/ [Accessed 14 August 2015].

Whiteside, A., 2009. *Is AIDS Exceptional?* AIDS2031 Working Paper No 25.

Whiteside, A. & Strauss, M., 2014. The End of AIDS: Possibility or Pipe Dream? A Tale of Transitions. *African Journal of AIDS Research*, 13(2), pp. 101–108.

Wilson, P., Wright, K. & Isbell, M., 2008. *Left Behind: Black America – A Neglected Priority in the Global AIDS Epidemic*. Los Angeles: Black AIDS Institute.

World Bank, 1999. *Confronting AIDS: Public Priorities in a Global Epidemic*. London: Oxford University Press for the World Bank.

World Health Organization, 2008. *Task Shifting: Rational Redistribution of Tasks among Health Workforce Teams: Global Recommendations and Guidelines*. Geneva: WHO.

World Health Organization, 2014. *HIV/AIDS Fact Sheet*. Geneva: UNAIDS.

World Health Organization, 2015a. *Guidelines on When to Start Antiretroviral Treatment and Pre-Exposure Prophylaxis for HIV*. Geneva: WHO.

World Health Organization, 2015b. *HIV/AIDS Fact Sheet Number 360*. Geneva: World Health Organization.

Wouters, E., Van Rensburg, H. & Meulemans, H., 2010. The National Strategic Plan of South Africa: What are the Prospects of Success after the Repeated Failure of Previous AIDS Policy? *Health Policy and Planning*, 25(3), pp. 171–185.

Wringe, A., Cataldo, F., Stevenson, N. & Fakoya, A., 2010. Delivering Comprehensive Home-based Care Programmes for HIV: A Review of Lessons Learned and Challenges ahead in the Era of Antiretroviral Therapy. *Health Policy Planning*, 25, pp. 352–362.

Yeboah, E., 2007. HIV/AIDS and the Construction of Sub-Saharan Africa: Heuristic Lessons from the Social Sciences for Policy. *Social Science & Medicine*, 64(5), pp. 1128–1150.

Young, I., 2015. Imagining Biosocial Communities: HIV, Risk and Gay and Bisexual Men in the North East of England. *European Journal of Cultural Studies*, 19(1), pp. 33–50.

Index

Note: Page numbers followed by "n" denote endnotes.

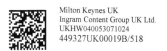